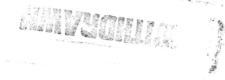

THE BEARDED GENTLEMAN

The Style Guide to Shaving Face

ALLAN PETERKIN & NICK BURNS

Arsenal Pulp Press | Vancouver

ARSENAL PULP PRESS
#102, 211 East Georgia Street
Vancouver, BC Canada V6A 1Z6
arsenalpulp.com

The publisher gratefully acknowledges the support of the Canada Council for the Arts and the British Columbia Arts Council for its publishing program, and the Government of Canada through the Book Publishing Industry Development Program and the Government of British Columbia through the Book Publishing Tax Credit Program for its publishing activities.

The authors and publisher assert that the information contained in this book is true and complete to the best of their knowledge. All recommendations are made without guarantee on the part of the authors and Arsenal Pulp Press. Readers may wish to contact their healthcare provider with specific health-related questions. The authors and publisher disclaim any liability in connection with the use of this information. For more information, contact the publisher.

Efforts have been made to locate copyright holders of source material wherever possible. The publisher welcomes hearing from any copyright holders of material used in this book who have not been contacted.

Cover design by Electra Design Group; cover photograph © Getty Images
Illustrations by Jaye Lyonns

Printed and bound in Canada on FSC-certified paper

Library and Archives Canada Cataloguing in Publication

Peterkin, Allan D.
        The bearded gentleman : the style guide to shaving face / Allan Peterkin & Nick Burns.

Includes bibliographical references and index.
ISBN 978-1-55152-343-9

    1. Beards. 2. Shaving. 3. Grooming for men.
I. Burns, Nick, 1980- II. Title.

RA777.8.P48 2010   646.7'044   C2010-901953-9

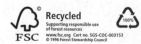

Recycled
Supporting responsible use
of forest resources
FSC
www.fsc.org Cert no. SGS-COC-003153
© 1996 Forest Stewardship Council

Acknowledgments

For Robert, Meg, Skip and Millie

Special thanks to Nick Burns for a wonderful, fun collaboration (and for his high-tech web-wizardry); to Brian, Robert, Shyla, Susan, and Janice at Arsenal Pulp and to Amanda Miller for help with the manuscript; and to Phil Olsen, Jay Della Valle, Eric Brown, and Dr Paul Cotterill (for their hair-raising tips) and to Dr Chris Moss and Brett and Kate McKay (for expertise on fur-removal). Thanks also to all the wonderful facial hair (and shaving) communities who keep things alive on their websites, blogs, and through their charity work.
—AP

My heartfelt thanks to Allan for his patience and genius during our fun collaboration; Mom, Dad, Pamela, Heather, Alex, and Cathy for their love and support; Susan, Shyla, Brian, Janice, and everyone at Arsenal Pulp Press for making this book possible.

Many thanks to everyone who contributed to the book, including Martial Vivot, Shorty Maniace, Brad Katchen, MD, Neil Sadick, MD, and the people behind the websites, books, and magazine articles that assisted us in our research.

Special thanks to Susan Rasky for her inspiration, editing brilliance, and guidance; Amanda Miller for her research; Aaron Krach and Sally Chew for lending their eyeballs; Chris Nutter of Nutter Media for his generous marketing support; Tyler Sipe for the great photos; Richard Koci Hernandez and Josh Williams for their help with *Beardedgentleman.com*; Paul Grabowicz, Jerry Monti, Bill Gannon, Neil Henry, and the entire Graduate School of Journalism at the University of California, Berkeley for all the support.
—NB

CONTENTS

Chapter Five: Saying Goodbye

CHAPTER ONE

SHOULD I SHAVE OR SHOULD I GROW?

One morning, you look in the mirror and it hits you. You basically like your face, but it's time for a change. (We're not talking plastic surgery.) You've always been Mr Clean-Cut. You're starting to look more and more like your dad (and nice as he is, that's not what you're aiming for). You're feeling like a corporate drone. Or maybe your trademark goatee is going grey and your dentist (who just charged you $933 for a filling) has the exact same growth on his chinny-chin-chin. You have a low-cost, all-empowering option, but it's time for a decision: You can either drop the razor or pick it up. And you don't have to ask anybody for permission (though everybody will have an opinion!).

Men just like you the world over now change their facial hair whenever they like, and for all kinds of reasons. You may want to look older (or younger), more laid-back and playful (or more macho), or show that you're in some kind of transition (think of Al Gore's beard after he lost the election, or the one on your recently divorced buddy).

Whatever your fuzzy (or clean-cut) motivation, this fine volume will help you pick a look, maintain or modify it, and then eradicate it (in style) so you can start all over. Beardies and Babyfaces unite! We are one and the same. Your face is your canvas—now go to town!

History 101: Why Men Grow Fuzz

Why have men grown (or removed) their facial hair?

The answer was fairly simple until the twentieth century. Cavemen really had no choice because shaving hadn't been invented. From the Neanderthals onward, once a guy hit puberty, something bristly started sprouting on his face. Shaving (or at least plucking hairs out with clamshells) began about 2,000 BCE. Thereafter, whether Egyptian, Greek, Roman, or Judeo-Christian, you had to grow a beard to indicate your religion, class, and allegiance to your king. You sometimes removed it if your clergyman told you it was Satanic (rather than saintly), or if, like Oscar Wilde, you rebelled and took it off (so as not to look like all those bushy Victorians). Mustaches were popular in the military, but aside from that, and depending on the time and place, could be interpreted as foppish, fiendish, or foreign. Basically, you took your cues from those in charge.

The twentieth century is when things really started to get interesting. King Camp Gillette started producing his disposable razor blade in 1903 and revolutionized shaving forever. After both world wars, men became convinced that clean-shavenness signified godliness, patriotism, and modern life. A male grooming industry was born, and razors (both blade and electric) with accompanying foams, tonics, and aftershaves became big business. Our fathers, grandfathers, and great-grandfathers wouldn't have been hired with beards and mustaches (unless they were orthodox clergy or university professors). Between 1900 and 1950, men were (apart from a few "commies" and mustachioed Hollywood types) essentially hairless, but thereafter every decade brought its own furry expressions. Western civilization increasingly began to trumpet individualism over communal identity. The fifties gave us beatnik beards, daddy-o Soul Patches, and Elvis sideburns. The sixties brought long-haired, wild-bearded hippies. The seventies brought swinger/bi/porn-star mustaches. The eighties brought designer stubble. Modern men were no longer taking their cues from politicians (who never have facial hair) and clergy

Why Men Grow Fuzz

Here are the twenty most common answers we got when we asked modern guys why they grow facial hair:

1. I hate shaving.

2. I want to look older (or younger).

3. I want to hide my double chin or facial scars.

4. I'm losing it up top (balding) and want to balance things out.

5. I'm leaving my marriage/relationship and it's time to put on a new face.

6. It's more masculine and people find it hot.

7. It's a family tradition.

8. I did it to drive my family crazy.

9. I admire Che Guevara, Fidel Castro, or any other number of left-wing politicians.

10. My favorite rock star/athlete/actor has one.

11. I'm changing my life and want to change my look.

12. I'm on holiday/hiatus.

13. It's my playoff/layoff/strike beard.

14. I'm grieving a loss.

15. Barring store-bought T-supplements, it's the only thing left that women can't do.

16. Guys can't wear makeup (most of the time), but we can use facial hair to highlight our features.

17. I grow one in the winter to stay warm.

18. I'm no corporate slave. I can get away with it at work.

19. It's natural/God-given.

20. It's fun, and I like the reactions I get.

(who usually don't) and instead looked to rock stars, movie actors, and athletes for what was cool, playful, and rebellious.

And then, all hell broke loose in the nineties. Grunge-rockers like Kurt Cobain started growing goatees and so did sports stars, boy bands, and brat-pack Hollywood types. Before you knew it, you and your dad (and your dentist) had one too. Workplaces (with the consistent exceptions of government and high finance) became more relaxed about facial hair, because everybody (including your boss) was proving that he was no corporate slave. Men took their cues from pop culture (rather than their *Mad Men* clean-shaven fathers or other authority figures), and their partners, for the most part, didn't seem to mind. Fussy metrosexuals soon gave way to bad-boy retrosexuals sporting playoff beards, mountain-man tufts, break-up beards, bear fur, and F-you beards.

If history has taught us anything, it is that facial-hair trends cycle on and off, but this modern interlude shows no signs of slowing down. All of the large shaver companies have seen the writing on the wall and have introduced products that allow you to clip within a millimeter of your life, so that you can combine stubble with a full stache (or embrace one of an endless number of partial beard combinations and permutations that you will find in the pages that follow). Every imaginable facial hair expression has been manifested since the 1990s, from full-on ZZ Top beards to micro-carved architectural experiments, from stubble with a full stache to a Soul Patch with a pencil-thin mustache, sideburns, and a chinstrap. It's all up to you.

Mathematically, the variations are endless. Fuzz now knows no bounds in terms of age, class, or race. (Even gender is up for grabs, as female-to-male transsexuals take testosterone and wear facial hair as a proud celebration of masculinity.) Surveys tell us that sixty percent of men in their twenties now sport some kind of facial hair. You know things are serious when razor and shaver companies start inventing products that allow for trimming and pruning rather than total removal.

The Hair That Makes the Man

Few matters of personal style carry more power—or create more controversy—than facial hair. Both beloved and reviled throughout history, we
believe that mustaches, beards, and sideburns deserve respect, for they
are the very essence of masculinity.

Facial hair styles fall in and out of social favor, not to mention fashion and political tastes, but they continue to withstand the test of time.
They've created sex symbols, yet just as emphatically have been rejected
as a sign of filth or moral failure. Certainly one thing is clear: The whiskers make the man!

Power Trip

Some of history's greatest leaders have adorned their faces with beards
and mustaches. Generals, philosophers, Nobel Prize winners, poet lau-
reates, presidents, emperors, kings, rock stars, and red carpet royalty all
have grown whiskers in glorious displays. However, an equally impressive
cast of villainous characters has also sported facial hair.

Whether the wearer is a hero or villain, sinner or saint, barbarian or
gentleman, a face full of fuzz has been repeatedly heralded as a sign of
dominance, wisdom, and virility. This may be in part because it reminds
us of men's early days on earth as hunters. But some also theorize that a
beard creates the appearance of a larger jaw and highlights the teeth as
potential weapons, making it a logical style choice for early humans who
were fighting off beasts in the wild.

In modern American politics, on the other hand, facial hair is considered a style faux pas. No serious presidential candidate has sported a
beard or mustache since William Howard Taft became the twenty-sev-
enth Commander-in-Chief in a Wild-West stache.

When Richard Nixon and John F. Kennedy engaged in the first-ever
televised political debate in 1960, even the hint of facial hair proved di-
sastrous for Nixon, whose sallow look and sloppy five o'clock shadow
were no match for JFK's golden tan, clean-shaven face, and preppy New
England style. Political experts say that single debate helped win the

election for the Senator from Massachusetts. The moral of the story is not that beards can undo one's career—but that unkempt facial hair can cripple just about any campaign.

The Rite of Passage

Teenage boys in the throes of puberty anticipate the sprouting of their first wiry whisker with almost as much excitement as the loss of their virginity—all the more thrilling as a rite of passage into manhood for kids who have watched their fathers perform the daily ritual of shaving.

Playwright, poet, and playboy William Shakespeare once wrote, "He that hath a beard is more than a youth, and he that hath no beard is less than a man." Indeed, the beard can even be viewed as a kind of bold advertisement of a man's readiness to have sex and procreate. It all starts at about the same time: as a boy's cheeks begin to sprout, his hormones are running wild with the first explorations of desire.

The Scientific Research

From an anatomical perspective, whiskers are a key facial feature that separates men from women; they grow in direct response to the presence of male hormones. Testosterone is converted into dihydrotestosterone, which acts like Miracle-Gro in the hair bulb.

Other scientific evidence that fur = machismo includes a study published in 1973 in the journal *Psychology* by psychologist Robert Pellegrini (and later confirmed by others). He concluded that "the male beard communicates an heroic image of the independent, sturdy and resourceful pioneer, ready, willing and able to do manly things." He arrived at this pro-beard conclusion by photographing eight men with various facial hair styles and asking subjects to rate specific personality traits. The most bearded among them earned the highest marks for being more masculine, dominant, intelligent, courageous, mature, confident, liberal, and healthy.

While one might think perceptions have changed since the 1970s, consider a more recent study published in the journal *Personality and*

The Pros and Cons of a Hairy Face

Pros:

keeps you warm

is easier on the skin than shaving

is less demanding to keep up than daily shaving (only partly true—read on!)

allows you to change your look

plays up facial strengths and disguises weaknesses

makes you look more masculine

is a personal expression

signifies rebellion, playfulness, freedom

reduces costs (i.e., no razor blades)

is a "natural way of being"

Cons:

is not maintenance-free; still requires upkeep

may turn off potential mates and may frighten small children

may lead to false assumptions about the integrity of your character and may prevent you from getting hired or promoted

may make you look like a late adapter/copycat or conformist (remember the pathetic middle-aged ponytail?) if you grow a popular beard style

the style you pick may not suit your face (unless you read on), so there's ample room for serious esthetic error

can be a safety risk if you need to wear a protective mask with a tight seal, i.e., during viral epidemics, gas attacks, or fires

your mom probably won't like it (although your dad might, but then he just might copy your style)

you may be stopped more often at customs, security desks, and airline counters

Individual Differences in 2008 by Nick Neave and Kerry Shields. The researchers asked sixty women between the ages of eighteen and forty-four to rate pictures of men's faces with different levels of beardedness on perceived traits of masculinity, dominance, attractiveness, and other qualities. While a face with "light stubble" was repeatedly picked as the most attractive, one with a "heavy beard" was labeled the most socially mature, masculine, and aggressive. The participants viewed a "light beard" as the most dominant and best for relationships—both long and short term. Nearly across the board, however, being "clean-shaven" was rated among the lowest in terms of dominance, attractiveness, masculinity, age, maturity, relationship desirability, and aggression.

Maybe now you'll think twice before picking up that razor and clearcutting your whiskers.

> **I would just like to say that it is my conviction**
> **That longer hair and other flamboyant affectations**
> **Of appearance are nothing more**
> **Than the male's emergence from his drab camouflage**
> **Into the gaudy plumage that is the birthright of his sex.**
> **There is a peculiar notion that elegant plumage**
> **And fine feathers are not proper for the male, when actually**
> **That is the way things are**
> **In most species.**
>
> —*"My Conviction," from* Hair *by James Rado and Gerome Ragni*

Changing Times, Changing Attitudes

No other period in recent history embraced hair more than the 1960s. The hippies, protesting against the Vietnam War, the draft, and all the clean-cut military ways, let it all hang out. Men and women in the rapture of "free love" went wild, cultivating hair into long, flowing locks. Unkempt bearded faces proliferated, and being hirsute was widely celebrated. Long locks and whiskers even took center stage on Broadway in the musical *Hair*.

By the 1970s, gay men revolted against the tired stereotype of being "feminine" and adopted a hypermasculine look of their own. Mustaches and beards paired with lumberjack plaid shirts, work boots, and tight jeans became de rigeur. Straight men (and porn stars and swingers) followed suit, and some of Hollywood's leading men adopted tough images replete with beards, goatees, and mustaches. As the decade came to a close, a new guard of hirsute manly icons emerged: think Shaft, Mr T, Tom Selleck, and Burt Reynolds.

But with fashions, what's in one day is out the next. As we all know, preppies and metrosexuals came along and cleared the facial landscape for a time. But the new millennium marked the return of the manly man, with the fur-style pendulum swinging to the other extreme.

In part, this change is because so many women began to tire of dating prepubescent plucked chickens and longed for the days of burly masculinity. And postmodern guys want to rebel, have fun, be sexy, and show that they're not corporate slaves—all with one furry swoop. Whatever the reason, facial hair is reclaiming its rightful place as sexy and cool.

Real men have hair.

Who Grows There?
What Facial Hair (or the Absence Thereof) Says About You

Your face is a blank canvas. You sprout something on it. In your mind, you look like Brad Pitt. You want to be playful, rebellious, liberated, erotic—but, alas, the world may not see you this way. How others read your face depends on their previous exposures to and associations with facial hair. Some will see Santa; others will see Satan. You are unlikely to be hired in government or finance, but your odds are good in information technology, creative fields, and academia. If you are of Middle Eastern descent and wear facial hair, the sad fact is that you are more likely to be stopped at customs or security checks at the airport. Your college co-ed neighbor might think you look hot, but your grandfather, remembering the Great Depression, will think you look like a bum. In short, the postmodern beard is up for grabs. Wear it proudly, but be prepared to be misunderstood.

What the Hell is Pogonophobia?

Pogonos (πώγων) is the Greek word for beard, and a phobia is a fear, dislike, or loathing of something. A lot of furry men believe that they are discriminated against in terms of employment, election to office, and mate selection and are targets of a lot of negative cultural projections because of their beards (such as that men wearing them are dirty, lazy horn dogs who can't be trusted). You can't judge a face by its fur cover, but lots of uninformed folks do. Take a stand for facial hair of all kinds! Check out the resources at the end of this book for beard-rights and activism organizations. We should all have the right to grow (or shave) with impunity!

The Beard Liberation Front (BLF) in Great Britain will tell you that bearded men are less likely to be hired and they have even conducted experiments to prove it. The organization sent men with the identical résumés on a job hunt, with or without facial hair, and those "without" were hired more often than their smooth-skinned counterparts. The BLF condemns prevalent pogonophobia, but attitudes are slow to change. Workplaces generally have the right to establish dress/appearance codes and insist that if you don't like it, you need not apply.

Three Famous Fuzz Devotees Tell Us What Their Facial Hair Has Taught Them

Lessons from three facial hair heroes.

Five Things I Have Learned from Wearing a Beard
by Phil Olsen

Phil Olsen is the founder and self-appointed captain of Beard Team USA, which competes for the United States at the biennial World Beard and Moustache Championships. He stumbled into the WBMC in Sweden in 1999 and noticed immediately that the USA was underrepresented. Since then he has striven to make the USA a powerhouse in international bearding and to transform the WBMC into a world-

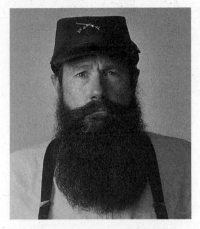
Phil Olsen photographed by Zach Ramey

class event worthy of its name. He is a semi-retired lawyer and part-time judge.

1. Some people think ZZ Top is a person rather than a band. I wish I had a dollar for every person who has asked me, "Are you ZZ Top?"
2. The worst thing about having a beard is not knowing when there is food in it. Real friends will let you know it's there.
3. Beards command respect among other men. Men often tell me, "I wish I had a beard like yours."
4. For every negative beard stereotype (Osama bin Laden, Rasputin, Attila the Hun), I can think of a positive one (Lincoln, Jesus, Santa, God).
5. Americans support the American beard team. The Germans think the World Beard and Moustache Championships should honor those who are best at conforming to a standard, but for Americans, facial hair is about nonconformity!

Five Things I Have Learned from Wearing a Mustache
by Jay Della Valle

Jay Della Valle, chairman emeritus of the American Mustache Institute (AMI) and one of the grandfathers of the modern-day mustache movement, is known principally for his acclaimed feature-length documentary, *The Glorius* [sic] *Mustache Challenge: A Film about the Under 30 Mustache*. Jay and his film have garnered the attention of media outlets all over the world, receiving coverage from *Good Morning America*, *The Today Show*, *Geraldo at Large*, and *The New York Times*. Jay

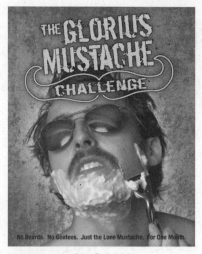

No Beards. No Goatees. Just the Lone Mustache. For One Month.

Image courtesy of Jay Della Valle

initiated the first-ever "mustache party rock 'n' roll tour" in April 2009 and his Stache Bash will be touring the US every April and November (see *gloriusmustache.com* and *stachebashevent.com* for details).

1. It's not the mustache that makes the man, it's the man that makes the mustache.
2. As the Spanish say, "A kiss without a mustache is like an egg without salt."
3. You can talk to other men with mustaches about mustaches, and they won't think that you're hitting on them or are some kind of swinger (or faded, chain-wearing porn star).
4. Stroking your stache in public creates the illusion that you can think deep thoughts and that you may be on the verge of saying something brilliant.
5. Once a mustache man, always a mustache man.

Five Things I Have Learned from Wearing Sideburns
by Eric Brown

Born and raised in California and now living in Jersey City, NJ, **Eric Brown** takes photographs and rides bicycles. In his spare time, he contemplates the future of competitive beard growing politics.

1. Zippers can be one hell of a challenge. Wintertime on the northeast coast mandates a jacket. Jackets have zippers. Zippers are the sworn enemy of long facial hair. One must lean forward to at least a forty-five-degree angle and gently coax the zipper up as the beard is continually brushed away from the zipper.

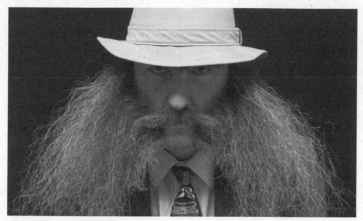

Self-portrait by Eric Harvey Brown

2. A "neck sweater" is a really handy thing in winter and isn't as uncomfortable in summer as you might think.

3. Blowing bubblegum is a really bad idea when you have sideburns.

4. Avoid barbecue ribs. Don't bring any food item which is wider than your mouth and covered in a thick sauce up to your mouth for a bite. Use cutlery instead.

5. People like to look (no, stare) at sideburns. Approvingly, disapprovingly, laughingly. Drunk people often shout about them from afar.

CHAPTER TWO

GET GROWING

The Perfect Fit: Facial Hair and Your Face

Deciding to grow facial hair is similar to planning a vacation; the look you settle on needs to suit your personality and style. Just as you wouldn't book a Caribbean cruise if you were afraid of the water, you shouldn't opt for a handlebar mustache if you're a pinstriped banker. Similarly, don't consider a style that makes your round face look rounder or your long face even more horse-like.

Before setting out on your facial hair expedition, take stock of your face shape, personality, the facial features you'd like to hide, your capacity to maintain a look, and any workplace rules you need to worry about. You might also want to consider the feelings and opinions of your significant other! While we agree that facial hair should be worn with great personal pride and individual enjoyment, don't forget that—with any luck—you won't be the only person enjoying it.

Identifying Your Face Shape

The first step in choosing the right beard or mustache style is determining your face shape and giving your facial features some thought. (Warning: this can be humbling, even painful at first.) Make a note of the strength of your jawline, the prominence of your cheekbones, the size of your lips, and the volume of your cheeks. All of these can affect which facial hairstyles will complement your look and which will have a nasty, adverse effect. Most styles can be tailored to suit your face shape, but the more you consider these factors, the better the fit.

While faces comes in all sorts of shapes and sizes, all are basically one of these three:

1. Round: A round face has soft features. Think fuller cheeks, hard-to-find cheekbones, and a soft jaw-line—maybe even a second chin. (Think Elmer Fudd.)

2. Square/Angular: The angular face is one that has high, strong cheek-bones, a square jaw, and, in most cases, a strong chin. You lucky devil!

3. Oval/ Long: A long, narrow face is considered oval. The jaw-line isn't especially pronounced, but it can include a strong chin.

How to Choose a Style

Choosing a style of facial hair is about achieving a fine-tuned balance between face and hair. If your face is round, select a style that will have a slimming effect. If your face is oval or particularly hollow, opt for a look that adds weight to your cheeks.

If your face is round: Choose a facial hair shape with strong lines, block shapes, and angles to balance out the curves. Sideburns can slim the face by adding vertical borders as long as they are kept trimmed to mini-mize bushiness. A squared-off goatee or a beard with shorter whiskers on the cheeks and longer whiskers on the chin and mustache can also add some geometric balance. Harvesting an even patch of five o'clock shadow can also slim down a full face.

If your face is angular or square: Angular faces can get away with just about any look—that's why they are the preferred face shape for models. However, some angular faces with particularly high cheekbones might have sunken-looking cheeks. If that describes your face, you can add more girth to your cheeks by growing a beard. Leave it longer in the cheek area and avoid any strong lines along the edges—in other words, allow some stray hairs to grow outside the lines. The idea is to create a natural-looking border. Sporting a five o'clock shadow is another great option for highlighting your facial features.

If your face is oval: Why the long face? No problem. With the right kind of facial hair, you can balance out your face's extra length. Choose a full beard that covers the lower half of your face; by dividing your face into two hemispheres, it will automatically bring your mug into proportion. Avoid styles with strong vertical lines such as long sideburns, chin-straps, and goatees. These will only emphasize the length of your face. Try a beard that's thicker on the cheeks to add some width, while leaving the mustache and the area around the chin a pinch shorter.

Size Matters

When choosing a facial hair style, consider the size of your facial features. If a man has a large nose, a pencil-thin mustache will look like a hairy mistake instead of a style statement. Similarly, a man with a tiny nose should avoid a big, bushy stache—unless he wishes to look like a walrus (in which case, we commend you!). The right style should complement your face without overpowering it or being overpowered by it. Here are some general guidelines:

If you've got large facial features (i.e., mouth, nose, eyes, and chin), go for a larger, bushier mustache or beard style. It will balance out your facial features and provide a softer look.

If you have a prominent nose, consider a larger, thicker mustache such as a Chevron, Painter's Brush, or Handlebar (see pages 58, 61, and 52), but steer clear of thinner designs.

A long, narrow face requires a narrow-to-medium-sized mustache that's not too heavy in length or design. Stick to shorter styles and skinnier lines, such as the Clark Gable, Chaplin, or Military staches. Stay away from styles with vertical lines—such as the Horseshoe—that will only highlight the length of your face.

If you've got an extra large mouth (think Aerosmith front man Steven Tyler), choose an angular style such as the Pyramid mustache (see page 62) that is narrow at the top and wide at the bottom. The variety in length and angles will minimize the size of your mouth.

Don't overpower a smallish mouth with a big, bushy mustache. Instead, go for a shorter style. Growing the stache a smidge past the corners of your mouth will make your mouth appear a bit larger.

If you've got a wide mouth with a big upper lip, consider a large, bushy mustache with a part that divides the mustache into two sections. Try on a Handlebar and invest in some quality wax to get it just right.

See the Resources section (see page 147) for three of our favorite facial hair try-on websites.

Ask the Expert: Martial Vivot

Acclaimed stylist and barber **Martial Vivot** knows the male face. As the owner of one of Manhattan's best grooming salons exclusively for men, he has been styling celebrities and Wall Street power brokers alike for over twenty-five years. Here he shares some additional expert advice on how to pick a facial hairstyle that suits your face shape, how to hide a double chin, and why you should avoid "strong lines."

Q. What do you like about facial hair?

A. Facial hair is a great way to change the appearance and structure of the face. If there is something you want to hide or balance on your face, growing a mustache or beard is the way to do it. Beards and mustaches are accessories, like jewelry.

Q. Are there particular facial hairstyles that suit certain face shapes?

A. You do need to make sure the shape of the beard or mustache complements your face. But there is always a way to adjust and balance the style according to your face shape and where you have less or more growth.

Q. What should a man consider before growing a beard?

A. Grow your beard for a week or so in order to see exactly where and
how it grows. You might see some patches where you don't have hair,
for instance, which might prevent you from growing a full beard or a
goatee.

Choose a style that reflects what you are trying to accomplish. There
are two ways to do a beard or facial hair: You can use it to balance
out your face and hide certain features, or you can make a statement
and look more edgy. For example, you'd generally want to give an
oval face a beard that is slightly fuller on the sides and not so long
on the chin to soften the oval shape. But if you want to make a
statement, you can exaggerate your face shape instead by leaving the
hair on the chin slightly longer.

Q. What if someone has a really round face?

A. I don't generally like very strong lines and borders on facial hair, but
I do think they can help make a round face look more square. They
accentuate the cheekbones and add structure to the face. It's all about
the geometry of the face. With a round face, you also want facial hair
that's shorter on the cheeks and longer on the chin. A shadow is also
a good option because it makes the face look skinnier.

Q. Do you have advice for someone with an angular- or square-shaped
face?

A. You can do whatever you want! Brad Pitt has that type of a square
face. Just have fun. Enjoy. You're handsome. You have the perfect
face shape. I would try to stay away from strong lines and play more
with shadow. If you want to soften the really strong angles of your
face, you can leave your beard a bit fuller.

Q. What's so bad about lines?

A. I hate lines (that is, precision-cut borders). I believe a beard should look completely natural. You want to control the thickness, not the lines. If the lines are too strong, it looks unnatural and forced.

Q. How do you recommend trimming and shaping a beard?

A. Blend it as much as possible. First decide where your beard will be the longest and then adjust the other areas to complement that part of the face. Once you determine how long you want your beard, trim it slightly shorter as you approach the area where you want to create a line. Then trimming it closer along the edge will soften the border.

If you want to maintain a short beard, mustache, or five o'clock shadow, you'll need to trim it more frequently, two to three times a week. If you have a longer beard, trimming and combing once a week will keep it looking great.

Q. What are some of the most common mistakes guys make with their facial hair choices?

A. It's the lines along the edge, of course. When you create a line beneath the chin, there are two ways to do it: straight across or rounded. I recommend following the line of the jaw. You want to draw the line where the skin on your neck meets the skin on your chin. That's where you want to start to blend the border of your beard. It's also great for concealing a double chin. If you have a round face, you don't want to make a round line beneath the chin; it will accentuate the double chin. Instead, aim for something more angular. The reverse would be true for a man with a more angular or square face.

Q. What about mustaches?

A. We are seeing more guys with mustaches. We went through a period of rough cuts with more texture and spikes, but now it's more elegant, softer. But if you want to play with that sort of mustache, you need the whole look that goes with it. It's a suit. If you wear some ornate, highly styled mustache and you are just out jogging in shorts and a t-shirt, you're not making any statement. Your facial hair should reflect and complement your style, not compete with it.

Stop Shaving: When, Where, How?

Planning a Beard

Virtual Photoshop experiments aside, what you think you'll see may not be what you get. Just as certain types of clothing work with particular body types, certain styles of facial hair go better with certain facial structures. As mentioned previously, things to consider when planning a new look include:

- facial shape (round, long, oval, triangular, boxy, etc.)
- texture, color of your facial hair, and
- how much hair you have on your head.

Pick up a few men's fashion or fitness magazines and choose a style you think will fit your face. Ask your barber for his take, too.

Pick Your Timing

It is probably best to start growing during a vacation, layoff, or summer holiday. Other socially sanctioned times to grow beards are when you are grieving a dead loved one or during hockey playoffs, or if you convince everyone you're doing it for charity. The thing to avoid is people remembering Jack Nicholson in *The Shining* when they see your face.

Simply stop shaving for the first four to six weeks. This will allow your beard to grow in naturally and give you a sense of its color, pattern, and rate of growth and will also eliminate the risk of you zealously over-trimming or producing bald spots. You need a bush before you can start pruning! During the early stages of growth, eyebrow pencils can be used to conceal uneven patches and define irregular borders. Various beard touch-up products also exist (see lists of product resources at end of book).

Be Patient

Resist picking up the razor—even if you get flak from those around you. You'll be itchy at the start. A little bit of baby oil or moisturizer helps with that. Review the various beard style recipes in Chapter Three. For your first trim, consider asking a barber or stylist to shape your beard, mustache, or goatee instead of trimming without supervision—and bring a photo! If you are going to do it yourself, proceed with caution.

We repeat: Do not shave at all for the first four to six weeks. Let your beard grow out naturally so you can see its density and growth patterns. The first two or three shaves should be performed extra cautiously, especially if your beard growth density is minimal. Once you've got a fuller face of fur, you will be able to trim more freely and with less anxiety. When your beard is suitably long, you may want to have your barber or stylist shave the boundaries and neckline.

When you start pruning, use short, deliberate strokes, keeping the surrounding skin taut. You can plot the boundaries of your new beard with an eyebrow pencil and then trim away from the pencil boundary, taking care not to trim deeper than the established boundary. Uneven or rough areas can be refined later, once the initial shaping is complete. Leave your cheek area natural, using tweezers to pluck hairs that stray above the boundary of growth (no harsh pruning lines, please). Itching is normal during the first several weeks. Wash and condition your beard in order to minimize skin irritation and to ensure your facial hair remains suitably clean and crumb-free. Use a beard conditioner (yes, such things exist—visit your drugstore shaving aisle) or a conditioner for the hair on your head to help smooth things out during the early growth phases.

Style Timeline for Age-Appropriate Growth

There's nothing more pathetic than a fifty-year-old trying to look eighteen or a pimply youth parading patchy caveman wisps. Here are some rough age-appropriate style calculations (adapted with permission from *beardstylings.com*):

Chinstrap: 16–20

Soul Patch: 17–39

Scruff: 18 and up

Goatee: 18–34

Goatee with stache: 19–49

Mustache: 21 and up

Full Beard: 25 and up

Mustache and Soul Patch: 23 and up

Mutton Chops: 32 and up

Mutton Chops with stache: 35 and up

For some reason, the *beardstyling*s folks are anti-sideburn and view them as hairstyle affiliates, so read on for more on sideburns. Our own view is that every face is different and you need to experiment and get honest feedback from those around you. Remember all those forty-plus guys with ponytails in the 1980s? Try to avoid the "pathetic-stab-at-lost youth" aura if you're getting on and the "too cool for school" schtick if you're young.

General Tips for Early Growth

Days seven to fourteen are the messiest stage of beard growth (past the cool-stubble window).

To avoid food-lodged-in-beard embarrassments, ask your best friend or partner to have a subtle cue ready for you at the dinner table. Use your napkin a lot while you get used to your beard!

Esquire magazine (October 2009) advises that, "Precision should not be a factor in facial-hair borders." This means ultra-manicured, architectural experiments are ill-advised.

As a general guideline, confidently worn stubble and tidy sideburns work best. This could change—check our website (*www.beardedgentleman.com*) for updates!

Questions and Answers for Beardies

Q. I've stopped shaving, and people are starting to feel free to make snide remarks. What should I do?

A. Don't take it personally; be playful and have a set response such as, "May the furry force be with you," and flash them a peace sign. Pregnant women have to deal with uninvited remarks about their bodies all the time (even the odd grope), and they learn to cope. You will too.

Q. I'm a teenager, and my beard is pretty wispy and pathetic. Should I just give up?

A. Absolutely not! Full beard-growth capacity is not reached until your twenties or thirties. Work with what's growing best for you now, such as sideburns or your mustache, and go with that.

Q. I'm job hunting. Should I shave?

A. This is a complex one. It depends on what kind of work you're seeking. Certain workplaces have prohibitions against facial hair, such as fire departments, where a beard can prevent a good seal with a facial mask (which could save your life), and employees may be asked to shave. Creative and academic fields are usually ok. High finance and government usually aren't. Find out about the company, and see if they employ any furry brethren. If you're going to keep your facial hair for the job interview, be sure to tidy it up, get a good hair cut, and wear it with pride.

Q. What factors affect how my facial hair experiment will look?

A. Three things determine how facial hair looks: genetics, your age, and the color of your facial hair. Be realistic about your growth and, when in doubt, ask your barber for honest feedback.

Q. How can I make my beard softer for kissing?

A. You can use beard conditioner, hair conditioner, or coconut oil, and let the beard grow longer. Longer hair tends to be softer and allows the whiskers to lay flat, whereas short whiskers stick straight out and have hard, sharp ends.

Q. Will dyeing make my beard look thicker?

A. That all depends. You should use dye that's one or two shades lighter than the hair on your head. If you have good, even growth, the dye might make your hair look thicker; however, wispy, patchy growth will likely look more pathetic.

Q. How long will it take to achieve a foot-long beard?

A. Facial hair grows about half an inch a month, so it will be approximately two years before you have the full enchilada.

Five Tips for a Fur-Favorable Diet

A healthy diet promotes health hair growth on your head and face. Although taking extra supplements won't fill in bald spots, *not* getting enough nutrients will certainly produce them. Make sure you get enough:

1. **Protein**: hair is made from protein. Healthy sources include chicken, lean beef, eggs, and vegetable proteins such as legumes.

2. **Carbohydrates**: if you go extra-low-carb, your hair will fall out. Go for fruits, vegetables, whole wheat breads, and pastas.

3. **Water**: hair will dry out and or break off if you are perpetually dehydrated.

4. **Fat**: especially "good" fats, such as omega-3s from fish sources, will keep your scalp and other body hair healthy.

5. **Micronutrients**: such as vitamin C, biotin, zinc, and iron are all hair growth co-factors. A balanced diet should provide them all, but a multivitamin isn't a bad idea if you typically eat on the run.

Q. I don't need to use sunscreen if I have facial hair, right?

A. Wrong. Facial hair offers only partial protection against the sun's harmful effects, including wrinkles, discoloration, and even skin cancer. Look for a light cream or spray-on product, and rub it over your whole face, beard included, as you used to when you were clean-shaven.

Q. I want to shave the whole thing off. Are there any risks?

A. Read on to find out how to comfortably and safely remove a beard or other facial hair expression. Think about this carefully. Some men experience regret when they shave and state that they no longer recognize their faces. Others describe something akin to phantom limb pain where they feel like they've lost a vital body part. Some men have been dumped after they've shaven their beards. Eleanor of Aquitaine dumped her French husband Louis VII after he shaved because he didn't look so hot clean-shaven. She then took up with Henry II, King of England, and gave him her dowry, which included a lot of land. Three hundred years of war ensued (you've never heard of the War of the Whiskers?). Let this be a warning!

Q. Both my dad and my dentist have goatees now. Should I lose my own?

A. Alas, facial hair has become so ubiquitous that late adapters abound. You can either embrace solidarity with your elders, or pick up some fashion and sports magazines and keep flipping the pages until you find a new look to call your own (until they steal that one, too).

Q. I'm a smoker. How do I get rid of stains on my beard?

A. The easiest and least yucky-tasting way to do this is to buy some

The Bearded Good in History: Top 5

God

Santa

Jesus

Uncle Sam

Abe Lincoln

The Bearded Bad in History: Top 5

Satan

Attila the Hun

Osama bin Laden

Rasputin

Vlad the Impaler

smoker's toothpaste, brush or massage it in, and then wash it off. No more yellow stains, and you'll be oh-so-minty fresh.

Better yet, why don't you stop smoking?

Q. I like to use various products from different beard-care lines—shampoo, conditioner, mustache wax. Will my face explode?

A. Manufacturers want you to believe that you have to use their entire skin care line from start to finish or some weird chemical reaction will happen. This is not the case. Find products that work for you and use them consistently (and in the right order).

Q. Beards are easy, right? I just let mine grow?

A. Wrong, wrong, wrong. Beards and other facial hair combos are a responsibility and need to be trimmed, clipped, plucked, and shaped on a regular basis. Designer stubble, for example, is probably more work than shaving every day. So unless you plan to be the perfect slob, get with the program and read on.

Q. My face is red, raw, and nicked every time I shave. Should I just give up?

A. Razor burn, cuts, and ingrown hairs are all the results of poor shaving technique, using the wrong products, and using the wrong tools (see Chapter Four for the right way to do things).

Q. Why aren't we seeing more mustaches?

A. If bearded men complain that they're discriminated against, their mustachioed counterparts probably face more. Historically, the mustache has been associated with the fop (an effeminate guy), the foreigner (a terrorist), or the fiend (the Devil). The 1970s, with all those chain-wearing porn stars, pushy swingers, and bi-curious disco fanatics, probably didn't help much, either. Do not let stache-bashing impede you, however. Grow up and grow on.

Q. Are beards still considered religious?

A. Going back to the days of the Greek gods, beards have been an important part of religious iconography, and key world religions still embrace facial hair as a sign of the believer. Muhammad instructed his followers to cut their mustaches and allow their beards to

Five Things Not to Say to a Man with a Beard

1. Do you get food trapped in that thing?

2. You look like Santa! (or Satan!)

3. Your spouse doesn't mind?

4. Have you lost your job?

5. What are you hiding?

Five Things Not to Say to a Man with a Mustache

1. On leave from the Village People, are we?

2. Twirl the tips for me!

3. Are you working as a lounge lizard these days?

4. Hey, Ron Jeremy! (or other porn star)

5. You look like a foreigner! (or fop! or fiend!)

grow. Any attempt to remove facial hair is seen as disobedience to Allah and the Prophet. Sikh men wear long hair with an unshorn beard as one of the signifiers of belief. Orthodox Jews and Hasids wear beards following the Old Testament instructions, "You shall not round the corners of your heads, neither shall you mar the corners of thy beard" (Lev. 19:26-28). Hindus and Buddhists often wear facial hair, but there are no precise instructions, and the ascetics in their traditions usually grew natural beards. Rastafarians grew dreadlocks and beards in deference to "the line of Judah." Christians have been more fickle about facial hair. Orthodox priests wear beards, and their Roman Catholic counterparts tend to be clean-shaven. Historically, the religiosity of facial hair has flip-flopped countless times (see the book *One Thousand Beards: A Cultural History of Facial Hair* for the whole story).

Q. Help! My facial hair and I are being discriminated against at work. Is there anything I can do?

A. There have been significant test cases regarding the right to wear facial hair in specific workplaces including the military. Sometimes the insistence on clean-shavenness in the workplace has been reversed on the grounds of religious freedom or when a man can prove a medical condition, that is, that shaving produces severe ingrown hair and infection, which are a health risk. Do some Internet research about the issue before you hire a lawyer and things get costly; many workplaces still generally have the right to insist on specific codes of appearance.

Q. Help! I've got a bald spot on my beard!

A. Some electric trimmers have a blending attachment, which will allow more selective trimming. Use it as directed. Another option is to use a waterproof eyebrow pencil or a beard touch-up product to fill in the gap.

Q. Is it true that facial hair grows faster in the winter?

A. Facial hair is the fastest growing hair on your body and, in fact, it does grow fastest in winter (an evolutionary advantage because skin needs more protection in cold weather).

Q. How low *should* I go?

A. Some men prefer a very sharp, distinct line at the jaw with no facial hair moving on to the neck. Others embrace the other extreme and have their neck hair join their chest hair, a rather simian expression. We prefer the *juste milieu*, about an inch above the Adam's apple.

Q. How low *can* I go?

A. How long your beard will go is predetermined genetically. Jack Passion, a multiple World Beard and Moustache Championship victor, calls this "terminal beard."

Q. What's a philtrum?

A. That's the space between the margin

Five Things Not to Say to a Man with Sideburns

1. Jolly good, old man!

2. Hey Elvis, shake that pelvis!

3. Where's your hog, dude?

4. They let you go to work like that?!

5. Do your chops get caught in your turtleneck?

of your upper lip and your nose. The height of your philtrum will determine how thick and bushy your mustache should be. For example, a big philtrum (too large a space) usually requires a disguise or concealment.

Q. What about eyebrows? Aren't they facial hair too?

A. Yes, technically your eyebrows are facial hair; however, we implore you to avoid outdated metrosexual trends of plucking, thinning, and shaping. Get your barber to tidy things up or remove your unibrow. Don't get fancy yourself.

Q. In keeping with the above question, aren't nose hairs and ear hairs also facial hair?

A. Yes, indeed. Sadly, these hairs grow with gusto (as does the hair on your back). Your barber can use blunt scissors to trim ear and nose hairs, or you can buy a special trimmer to use at home. Nose and ear hairs are the only facial hair that should be discouraged—no, eradicated.

Q. Are any facial hair styles taboo?

A. Various styles come and go. Although certain styles are a matter of judgment, the only growth that remains taboo because of its obvious historical associations is the Hitler mustache. The style was benign when worn by Charlie Chaplin, but you simply can't wear it nowadays without the Nazi connection being made. No, it's not funny.

Q. Can my facial hair make me any money?

Five Myths About Facial Hair and Shaving

1. **Shaving will make hair grow faster and/or thicker.** Nice try. Facial hair is dead. It just seems thicker when it's short. When you shave a hair, the once-fine point becomes a blunt end, which feels thicker to the touch.

2. **You can judge a man by his facial hair.** Historically, this was true. You could tell a guy's affiliations, beliefs, loyalties, and social class by the presence or absence of fur on his face. Nowadays, a guy could look like Colonel Sanders and be a bastard or be a dead-ringer for Satan and be a pussycat.

3. **Shaving is bad for your skin.** Read on. If you do it right, it actually helps to exfoliate and keep the skin youthful (and oh-so-nice to touch).

4. **Plucking gray hairs from your beard will help more come back in their place.** Pure superstition. You can pluck away, but why not embrace your inner Santa?

5. **Beards keep growing after death.** We repeat: facial hair is dead. When you're dead, everything is dead. However, after you die, the skin shrinks and retracts, and this might make your beard look longer.

A. It was recently discovered that police officers in India were paid extra if they grew a mustache because it made them look tougher, more daunting, militaristic, and in charge. It's a very long shot, but you could ask your employer if you can get a fur allowance, premium, or raise. You can also contact manufacturers of facial hair products, razors, and shavers to see if they're looking for paid guinea pigs for new products. Entering contests is also an option (see Resources).

Q. Is it true that barbers used to draw blood, pull teeth, and do minor surgery?

A. This is absolutely true, which is why the original barber's pole had a brass bowl that housed leeches for bloodletting. White stripes signified clean bandages and the red, blood. The modern pole has a third blue stripe, which some say signifies dusky venous blood. However, barbers stopped doing all this medical stuff by the eighteenth century when surgeons took control of medical procedures.

Q. Can women grow beards?

A. There have always been bearded ladies, and a medical condition called polycystic ovary syndrome often leads to hirsutism, or excess facial hair on women. And in our age of millennial gender-bending, transsexual women transitioning will take testosterone to develop secondary male characteristics, including beards and mustaches.

Q. Will growing a beard make me smarter?

A. Some of the greatest brains in history, from Plato to Leonardo da Vinci to Freud, had nice beards. Alas, growing a beard might make you look more intelligent and mature, but unless you've got a high IQ, you'll just be a pretender (just as Elvis sideburns won't make you more musical or a pencil-thin mustache won't make you more suave).

Q. How can I have more fun with my beard?

A. Take a cue from pirates, ancient Gauls, and kids on campuses worldwide. Dye your beard metallic gold or cherry red. Braid it. Bead it. Separate it into pig-tails with rubber bands.

If you really want a conversation starter, shave off half, or have your right side longer than your left!

Ask the Expert: Paul C. Cotterill

So you want to grow a beard or mustache, but you're feeling follicularly challenged. Perhaps you dream of a face full of fuzz like a nice manicured lawn, but instead it grows more like weeds between the cracks in the sidewalk. You're not alone. Many men complain of patchiness or sparse growth getting in the way of their hirsute pursuits. Luckily, there are some things you can do that don't include fake mustaches or Halloween makeup.

We turned to **Paul C. Cotterill,** BSc, MD, ABHR, a Diplomate of the American Board of Hair Restoration Surgery and Past President, International Society of Hair Restoration Surgery, for answers. (See *DrCotterill.com*.)

Q. Are transplants successful for patchy facial hair growth? And what's a ballpark cost?

A. Yes, transplants are an option and can be successful. Generally, the hair is taken from the back of the scalp as a strip excision. A newer technique called follicular unit extraction (FUE) can also be utilized whereby one or two hair follicles at a time are removed from, in addition to the back of the scalp, other body areas such as the chest or back. Keep in mind that the newly transplanted facial hair will grow at the same rate and have the same texture as where it was taken from. Cost can range from $4,500 to $9,000, depending on length of the sessions and area covered. This treatment does not promise a thick, full beard but rather provides a light coverage of facial hair. So transplants can be very good for filling in patches of thin or no hair, rather than creating an entire beard in a completely hairless face.

Q. Is there any documented evidence that Rogaine (minoxidil), injected corticosteroids, red LED light, or laser combs can assist facial hair growth?

A. Injected corticosteroids will not help facial hair growth if the cause is genetically sparse facial hair (wispy growth). If the cause is alopecia areata (spot baldness) on the face, which is rare, it can, in many instances, respond to corticosteroid injections. The physician needs to be on the lookout for irregular or circular areas of total loss. There can be a family history of alopecia areata, and there may be other areas of the body affected, and/or a history of previous areas of alopecia areata. This type of patient is usually not a candidate for transplants as the newly transplanted hair may fall out. Genetically sparse facial hair (thin or patchy growth) will accept transplanted hair onto the beard area, and it will grow.

I do not know of any specific studies of minoxidil or low-level light lasers/laser combs assisting facial hair growth, but, theoretically, they could help. The newer version of minoxidil, which comes as a five-percent topical foam with glycerin as its base, is better absorbed and has less irritating qualities than the previous liquid spray forms using isopropyl alcohol as the base. So, if used, this would be off-label, with no guarantee of success. Patients should read the side effects pamphlet for the preparation before trying it. If someone is intent on trying it, I would suggest five percent topical minoxidil foam applied once per day. The laser comb products would be more difficult to use on the face because of the way they are designed.

Q. Are there any other treatments you would recommend?

A. Latisse (bimatoprost ophthalmic solution, 0.03 percent) is a prostaglandin analog. It is a prescription treatment for hypotrichosis (sparse growth) of the eyelashes. It increases growth—including length, thickness, and darkness. It has FDA approval and went on the market in the US in 2008. Bimatoprost ophthalmic solution has been on the market for many years as Lumigan, used for lowering intraocular pressure (IOP). An unexpected side effect was longer darker eyelashes.

There have been anecdotal reports of Latisse helping eyebrow regrowth. Whether this medication will help on the scalp or face remains to be seen, as adequate studies have not been performed and early results are not hopeful, likely due to the thickness of the skin on the scalp and face. However, future studies in this area and resulting products may lead to a prostaglandin analog that may help facial hair.

Five Most Popular Beards of the Twenty-first Century

(reprinted with permission from: *beardcoach.com*)

Number 5: The Natural

Covers the cheeks, chin, and upper lip; grown to a length of three inches or more.

Number 4: The Closely Cropped Full Beard

Between one-quarter to one inch of tidy growth, covering cheeks, chin, and upper lip.

Number 3: The Stubble Look

Between a beard and a five o'clock shadow, this stubbly style could also be known as the Weekender.

Number 2: The Van Dyke

A partial beard consisting of chin growth (a.k.a. a goatee) that connects to a mustache.

Number 1: The Urban Beard

A fine line of hair tracing the jawline, connecting to a finely trimmed mustache and fading to cropped sideburns at the hairline.

CHAPTER THREE

STYLING TIPS

An Illustrated Guide to Sideburns, Staches, Beards, and Everything in Between

Current Hot-off-the-Press Trends

With respect to facial hair combinations, colors, and length of growth, practically anything goes, but a few trends are worthy of mention.

In 2008, when writers in the entertainment industry went on strike, a phenomenon known as the "strike beard" was worn by celebrities such as David Letterman and Conan O'Brien as an act of solidarity for the undervalued, underpaid scribes of Hollywood.

Another fun trend is the "playoff beard," a superstitious practice started in the National Hockey League in which players drop their razors during the Stanley Cup playoffs and don't shave until their team is either eliminated or wins the cup. The trend goes back to the 1980s and the New York Islanders, but has become especially popular in the last ten to fifteen years, and has spread to other sports including football, basketball, and tennis.

An offshoot is the "fan beard," where fans of particular teams similarly grow facial hair while their favorite team is in the playoffs. Fans show their allegiance on their faces and have a lot of fun doing so.

The 2008 stock market crash led to the "layoff beard," which isn't as much fun. Men who lost considerable amounts of money stopped shaving out of despondency, fatigue or nihilism, much as men did during the Great Depression. Speaking of job-loss beards, Al Gore grew one after losing the presidential election in 2000 to George W. Bush. Gore was likely mourning his loss, changing his public face, and was also becoming an academic at Columbia University, where beards grow free. (The "breakup beard" is another example of a man changing his public face after experiencing a loss, in this case, of a relationship.)

The "band beard" is another trend where talented and not-so-talented musicians sprout unruly facial hair, make a lot of noise, and hope for a big contract. A less successful example was the "boy-band beard" such as that grown by A.J. McLean with his pencil-fine carvings when he was a member of the Backstreet Boys.

Finally, the "F-you beard" serves precisely the purpose it suggests.

THE BEARDED GENTLEMAN MANIFESTO

You are a man with testosterone in your veins. It is your right to grow facial hair as you see fit.

Never apologize, never explain. People will project all kinds of meaning onto your furry face. Let them. Then flash them a big smile.

Hold your head high—your fuzz will show better. Be fearless. Be playful. Whiskered confidence is sexy.

Defend the rights of your fellow facial-hair proponents. Challenge pogonophobia in all its forms.

Respect the shorn—they have not yet found their way.

Remember the proud history of facial hair throughout human development. At times it is seemingly vanquished only to sprout again, ever bushier.

You are no corporate slave. Push the whisker-envelope at work to pave the way for the next generation of furry faces.

Potential lovers only think they don't like facial hair. They need to be bewitched.

Change is good. Combinations of three simple ingredients—beards, staches, sideburns—are endless. Your face is your canvas to adorn.

Celebrate the hundreds of hours, the gallons of water, the thousands of dollars (in products) you have not wasted in shaving your face completely clean every single day of your life!

The Step-by-Step Style Guide to Mustaches

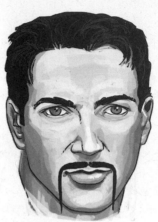

THE FU MANCHU MUSTACHE
A more dramatic version of the
Horseshoe mustache (see page 57).
Associated with a fictional character
from the popular twentieth-century
novels by Sax Rohmer—and later
in comics, television, and film—the
style maintains a slightly villainous
association because of its pop-cultural
history.

The Fu Manchu frames the mouth
with a similar shape as the horseshoe. However, it achieves that same effect with drooping whiskers that grow long from just below the corners of the mouth. The longer one grows the drooping tendrils, the more dramatic the effect.

How to achieve this style:

Shave your cheeks and chin clean while leaving the whiskers above the lip and just below the corners of the mouth untouched.

With an electric or wet razor, shave the outermost edges of your mustache into a downward slope, following the natural shape of the mouth to create a framing effect.

Use facial hair scissors to trim the whiskers above your mouth flush with the upper lip.

Hair at the corner of the mouth should be allowed to grow. It will take some time to cultivate adequate length for the whiskers to extend beyond your chin.

Use mustache wax to define the shape and create a more pointed, polished, or even sinister look.

MILITARY MUSTACHE
(also known as the Cop Stache)
Perhaps one of the most popular styles
of mustache is the Military or Cop
stache. You'll know it as the favorite
style among facial hair icons Tom
Selleck and Burt Reynolds, although
both gentlemen occasionally opted for
longer versions that bordered on the
Chevron style (see page 58).

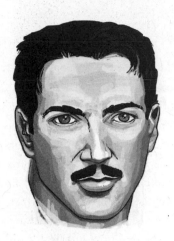

According to US Navy regulations,
a mustache must not extend below the
lip line of the upper lip. The width of
the stache cannot extend more than a
quarter of an inch horizontally beyond the corners of the mouth.

The Marine Corps, Air Force, and Coast Guard are slightly more
strict and require that a mustache not extend beyond the corners of the
mouth horizontally or vertically, and should not conceal any part of the
upper lip. These regulations are said to restrict facial hair so greatly as to
discourage its growth. Adjust them as you like, unless, of course, your job
adheres to similar regulations.

Both the Navy and Marines limit the length of individual whiskers to
just half of an inch or less—requiring rather fastidious grooming.

How to achieve this style:

Shave all facial hair on your cheeks, chin, and neck, leaving the mustache intact.

Use an electric or wet razor to remove any mustache whiskers that extend beyond the
corners of your mouth—or a quarter of an inch beyond, depending on which branch of
service you prefer.

With scissors and a narrow comb, trim the bottom of the stache until you have a strong
lower edge that is flush with the uppermost border of your upper lip.

Using a facial hair trimmer or scissors and comb, trim all whiskers to a uniform length of
half an inch or less.

HANDLEBAR MUSTACHE
(also known as the Howie or
the Wild West)

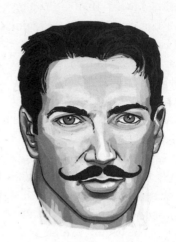

A classic style reminiscent of the
Wild West and certain members
of the Baseball Hall of Fame, most
notably Rollie Fingers. Many people
confuse the Horseshoe (see page 57)
with the Handlebar, likely due to the
association of the Horseshoe with
bikers.

The Handlebar style is similar to
the Fu Manchu, except the ends curl
up in small flourishes instead of drooping down. It's also thicker, and the
growth is fuller. This style requires some dedication to daily upkeep with
mustache wax and a comb.

How to achieve this style:

Following the line of your upper lip, shave the mustache into a downward slope from the
middle of your nose to the corners of your mouth, leaving a finger's width of hair.

The outer regions of the mustache require extra length in order to achieve the proper curled
appearance, so be patient.

Using mustache wax and a comb, draw a part in the middle of the mustache (if desired)
and sweep each section outward toward the corner of your mouth. If creating a part is too
difficult because your hair is too short or stubborn to hold the style, use a straight razor to
carve a narrow line in the middle to achieve the same effect.

With a bit more wax, carefully curl the edges of the mustache upward to your liking.

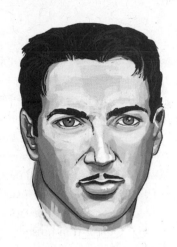

THE CLARK GABLE MUSTACHE

Once heralded as the King of Hollywood, Clark Gable, was one of the biggest sex symbols of all time and remains in the facial hair hall of fame for his short, thin mustache. The style requires strong, diagonal lines from the nose to the corner of the mouth with a similarly strong line creating a lower boundary. The mustache has a well-defined part in the center, following the natural crease between the lip and nose. Short styles like this one require daily maintenance. (Frankly, my dear, you should give a damn.)

How to achieve this style:

Your face should be clean-shaven, leaving only the mustache whiskers intact.

Using an electric shaver, trim your mustache hair to a length of approximately a quarter of an inch.

Trim away any mustache whiskers that progress beyond the corners of your mouth.

Beginning in the center and beneath the nose, trim each side in a diagonal line that passes sharply from your nose to the corner of your mouth.

Use a safety razor to shave clean the vertical crease running from the base of your nose to the upper lip.

Trim the lower mustache edge, forming a clean straight line.

THE PENCIL-THIN MUSTACHE

(also known as the Mouthbrow)

This style looks just like it sounds: a thin line of hair above the upper lip. It can be worn in many shapes and designs, from a Chevron-like angle to just a line that traces the upper lip. Perhaps the most notable Pencil-thin mustache today belongs to movie director John Waters.

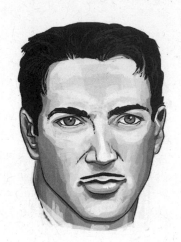

How to achieve this style:

For an angled look:

Shave your cheeks, chin, and neck clean; leave the mustache untouched.

With an electric shaver, trim your mustache whiskers to a uniform length of a quarter-inch.

Use a razor to shave a sharp, diagonal line from your nose to the corners of your mouth.

Repeat the last step, about an eighth to a quarter of an inch below the first line. This should create a quarter-inch width of hair running from your nose to the corner of your mouth.

Use an eyebrow pencil (yes, it's makeup) to fill in sparse areas or styling mishaps.

For the lip liner look:

Shave your cheeks, chin, and neck clean, leaving the mustache untouched.

With an electric razor, shave all remaining hair to a quarter-inch in length or shorter.

Using a razor to shave away all whiskers except for a quarter-inch line along the uppermost line of your lip.

Snip away any stray hairs that droop below the lip line with a pair of scissors.

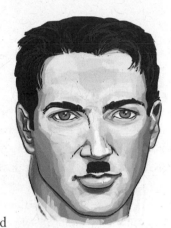

THE CHAPLIN MUSTACHE
(also known as the Toothbrush)
Comedic genius and silent film star Charlie Chaplin left his mark on the hearts and minds of moviegoers, but it's his trademark mustache that will live on eternally. His most memorable mustachioed character became famous in *The Tramp*, which opened in 1915. He sported a short, one-and-a-half-inch wide mustache with bold boundaries. Unfortunately, this particular facial hairstyle is marred by its association with Adolph Hitler, who adopted the same style during his rule of Germany from 1933 to 1945, thereby ruining a perfectly great mustache for the rest of us.

How to achieve this style:

As for the previous styles, your cheeks and chin are clean-shaven.

With a razor, shave the right and left sides of your mustache to leave a finger width of hair with defined edges on either side of your lip crease.

Use a pair of scissors to trim the whiskers flush with your upper lip edge.

With a razor, create a strong upper border between the mustache and your nose.

Trim between your nostrils and the upper mustache edge to form a clean line.

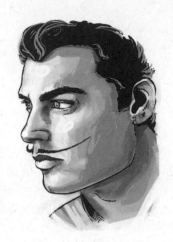

THE DALI MUSTACHE

Famed surrealist painter Salvador Dali didn't limit his bold style to the canvas. His long, pointed mustache not only defied conventional style in his day—it also defied gravity. It pointed upward and outward in long, twisted tendrils. Tamer variations on the style, in which the upward spikes are shorter and more restrained, are known as the Mistletoe or the Strip-teaser.

How to achieve this style:

Shave chin and cheeks, leaving the upper mustache whiskers intact to a point extending slightly beyond the outer edge of your lip.

Trim the centermost areas of your mustache until they're relatively short, using scissors.

Allow the whiskers closer to the corners of your mouth to grow long.

The outermost whiskers at the corners of your mouth are grown long enough to mold them into gravity-defying tendrils. Apply stiff wax sparingly and work it into the entire mustache.

Sculpt long points upward from each corner of the mouth and allow the wax to dry completely. Start sketching droopy, melting clocks in your spare time.

THE HORSESHOE MUSTACHE

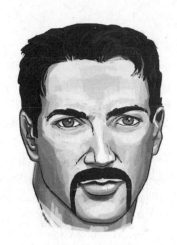

One of the most common styles of the 1990s, the Horseshoe mustache wraps around the mouth like an upside-down horseshoe, spanning the upper lip before extending down to the chin. The style is great for people with round or angular faces, but is not recommended for people with long or oval faces because it will accentuate a long face. Men with round faces should minimize the round shape of the horseshoe above the lip and opt for a more squared-off, block design. People often call the Horseshoe mustache a Handlebar (probably due to its popularity among bikers) but they are thoroughly mistaken.

As an alternative, the Horseshoe can also be worn upside-down (i.e., as a beard), beginning at the corners of the mouth and curving down to the chin, leaving the mustache area bare.

How to achieve this style:

Shave your cheeks clean, leaving the mustache, chin, and area surrounding the mouth untouched.

Using a razor, create a vertical line of hair (about half an inch wide) from the corner of your mouth to your chin. Do the same on both sides, paying close attention to keeping them even.

Using a razor, shave the upper edge of your mustache to create a sharp border, leaving just half an inch of hair. The hair should create a continuous horseshoe shape from above your lip to your chin.

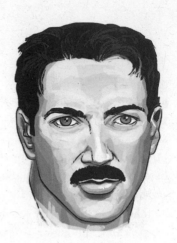

THE CHEVRON MUSTACHE

A fuller take on the Military Mustache (see page 51) with a sharper, angled design, the Chevron is grown full and slightly wider than the military version. It may conceal a bit of the upper lip, which makes it a little less food-friendly—unless you're the kind of guy who needs help straining his soup. The Chevron has a strong, angular and pointed shape that begins at the middle of the nose and extends beyond the corners of the mouth. If it reminds you of a certain bygone era, that's because this style peaked in popularity with Tom Selleck (Magnum, P.I.) in the late '70s and early 1980s.

How to achieve this style:

Shave your cheeks and chin clean, but leave the mustache untouched.

With a razor, shave a strong, diagonal line from your nose to a point about a quarter of an inch beyond the corner of your mouth.

Using scissors, trim any long stray hairs along your upper lip so the mustache is flush with the lip.

Allow your mustache to grow for a few weeks to achieve proper fullness.

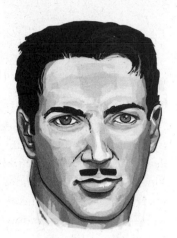

THE BUTTONS MUSTACHE

Similar to the Chaplin (see page 55), the Buttons style includes two identical small patches on each side of the lip crease. These don't extend past the corners of the mouth and are divided by a clear gap at the middle of the face. The boxy style works well for almost any face shape and provides a handsome—and politically correct—alternative to the Chaplin style that remains mired in historical controversy.

How to achieve this style:

Shave your cheeks and chin clean.

Using an electric shaver, trim mustache whiskers to about half an inch in length.

With a razor, create two identical, rectangular patches on both sides of the lip crease. Shave away the hair on the top and sides, leaving patches that are about half an inch in height and one to one-and-a-half inches in width. The total width should not extend beyond the corners of your mouth.

Remove hair from the lip crease to create a defined part between the two rectangular patches.

Perform regular maintenance a few times each week, as the look depends on its ultra-carefully styled appearance.

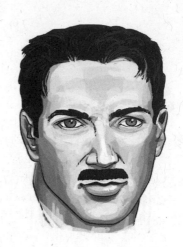

THE LAMPSHADE MUSTACHE

Another classic style with a descriptive title that says it all. The Lampshade is similar to the Chaplin (see page 55) but is narrower at the nose and wider at the lip. It features strong borders and carefully trimmed upper and lower boundaries as well. The hairstyle can be shaped with angled, vertical lines or—for a more romantic design—curved ones.

Don't get this style confused with the Pyramid stache (see page 62), which has more extreme angles between the top and bottom.

How to achieve this style:

Shave your chin, cheeks, and neck, leaving the mustache area untouched.

Use an electric trimmer to shave the mustache whiskers down to a quarter to half an inch in length to create a clean-cut and controlled look.

Using a straight razor or outliner, create an angled border on the left and right sides. Try to keep the angle around forty-five degrees. Most importantly, both sides should be angled evenly. Any tiny mistake will surely become a glaring one!

A straight razor or outliner can also create a clean line at the top and bottom of the mustache. The style shouldn't cross over the lip line or reach up to your nostrils.

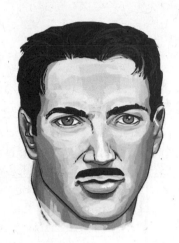

THE PAINTER'S BRUSH MUSTACHE

This style should be considered a Walrus (see page 63) for beginners. Similar in shape, it's worn much shorter and doesn't cover the mouth. In fact, one can easily grow a Walrus mustache from a Painter's Brush. The Painter's Brush resembles both an artist's brush and a brush stroke. It's worn short, extending the full width of the lip with slightly rounded corners and upper boundary.

The rounded corners of this style make it an unflattering choice for men with round faces, for whom the angled shape of a Chevron might make a better choice.

How to achieve this style:

Shave your cheeks, chin, and neck as usual, leaving the mustache area untouched.

Use an electric trimmer to cut the stache whiskers to between a quarter and a half inch in length.

With an outliner or razor, create a slightly rounded edge at the outermost corners and the top of the mustache.

Use a pair of scissors or an outliner to trim whiskers along the lower edge so they are flush with your lip line.

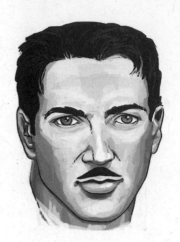

THE PYRAMID MUSTACHE

This style has a number of variations in design, but the basic shape is always the same. It begins with a wide base at the lip and tapers up to a near point under the nose. It is similar to the Lampshade (see page 60), but with sharper angles.

How to achieve this style:

Shave your cheeks, chin, and neck, while leaving the mustache untouched.

Use an electric trimmer to cut the mustache whiskers to about a quarter-inch in length.

With an outliner or razor, create a sloped border that starts at the middle of your nose and extends to the corner of your mouth. If feeling particularly adventurous and skilled, you can create a more curved design.

Repeat the last step on the other side of the mustache. Make sure both sides are even and equally sloped. Each side should be a mirror image of the other.

With facial hair scissors or an outliner, trim the lower edge of the mustache to prevent whiskers from crossing the lip line.

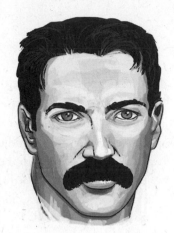

THE WALRUS

Like the one worn by the charming beast it's named after, this long mustache droops over the lips and covers part of the mouth. While this particular look could make eating certain foods difficult, it's certainly unforgettable. The style is grown similarly to the Painter's Brush (see page 61), but is taken to a longer extreme.

How to achieve this style:

Shave your cheeks, chin, and neck, leaving the upper lip area untouched.

Grow out your mustache for several weeks.

Brush the whiskers downward to cover your upper lip and part of your mouth.

Using a pair of scissors and a comb, trim the lower edge of the mustache so it appears even.

Buy a mustache cup—a special sippy-cup-like mug that protects your mustache from liquids. Or avoid foamy drinks and soups and wash your mustache at least once every day.

THE ENGLISH

Not just reserved for gentlemen with a British pedigree, this stache offers an air of old-world sophistication. It is a full mustache parted in the middle and combed to the sides. The outer regions are twisted and styled with wax to extend horizontally from the face—sometimes with a slight lift on the ends.

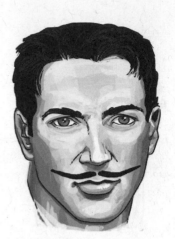

How to achieve this style:

Shave your cheeks, chin, and neck, leaving the beard area untouched.

Shave whiskers to about a quarter of an inch beyond the corners of your mouth.

Allow your mustache to grow long enough to style with a comb. This could take months, so be patient. The outer regions of the mustache, near the corners of the mouth, will require the longest whiskers.

Using a comb, part the mustache in the middle and sweep each section outward toward the corners of the mouth.

Work a pea-sized amount of mustache wax into the long whiskers and begin to gently twist them, moving from the base to the tip.

If you want to create a more defined part in the style, use a razor to shave away the hair within the lip crease.

The Step-by-Step Style Guide to Beards (and Partial Beards)

THE SHORT BOXED BEARD

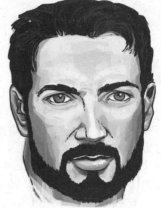

A short boxed beard looks carefully sculpted and groomed thanks to its close crop and defined borders. The whiskers are limited to the cheeks, upper lip, and chin and extend just an inch or two beneath the chin. Not only does this style highlight your cheekbones, but it also emphasizes the jawline (even if yours appears a tad weak) and can camouflage a second (or third) chin.

Because it relies on your own beard's natural shape, it can complement any face shape from angular and oval to heart-shaped and round.

How to achieve this style:

Using a razor, shave away the stray whiskers from the less dense areas of your cheeks. This will highlight cheekbones and other bone structure.

Using the natural borders of your beard growth as a guide, create a sloping border from your sideburn to the mustache. The key is to remove as few whiskers as possible to keep regular maintenance to a minimum.

Repeat the last step on the other side of your face. Try to maintain a balance between both sides of your face so the beard appears symmetrical.

To create a lower border, allow the beard to grow about one to two inches beneath your jawbone and remove any hair below that line with a razor. You can create a more natural-looking line by trimming the hair along the border a tiny bit shorter to blend away the strong line. (If you want to camouflage a second chin, follow the natural border where your chin meets your neck.)

Use a beard trimmer, clipper, and/or razor two to three times a week to maintain the borders and length. The color and density of your beard will determine its ideal length. Trimming to a quarter of an inch is a good start. Dark beards tend to look fuller than light whiskers. If your beard is blonde or red, allow it to grow a little longer to appear full and filled in.

THE POET'S BEARD

A favorite among college students who can't cultivate a full beard, the Poet's Beard is a derivative of the goatee. It is kept short and occupies three to four inches of space below the chin. It is usually coupled with a Soul Patch (see page 74) to increase credibility as an artist.

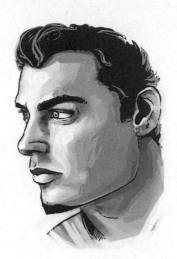

How to achieve this style:

Shave your cheeks, upper lip, throat, and the area immediately below the lower lip.

Leave intact the hair at the point of your chin and extending a short length along the jawline.

Using a razor, form a defined edge that blends along the jawline into the thicker chin hair.

Trim the beard to a short, blunt point. Look thoughtful and forlorn.

Quick Tip: If your beard becomes unbearably itchy on your neck or chin, it's likely caused by the whiskers under your chin brushing against those on your neck. As a remedy, trim or shave the hair on your neck. If your face feels itchy, apply a moisturizer, aloe gel, or low-potency (over-the-counter) cortisone cream to the area for immediate relief.

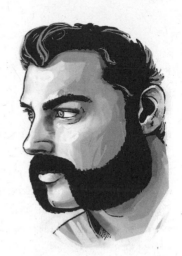

THE FRANZ JOSEF BEARD

Named for the nineteenth-century Austrian Emperor who sported a unique beard, the style consists of overgrown and highly cultivated whiskers growing on the cheeks, side-burns, and mustache. The mustache is the only area that bridges the divide between the left and right sides of the face. The chin, neck, and the area below the chin are left barren. It's a bold and unforgettable style fit for an emperor. The twentieth-century Grand-Duke Alexei Alexandrovich of Russia also adopted the look.

After three to four weeks of growth, you'll be ready to set the foundation for this distinguished style.

How to achieve this style:

Shave your cheeks in a slope extending from the sideburns to the outermost tips of the mustache.

Shave your chin and below your lower lip to create a sharp line of whiskers that form an arc over the upper lip.

Following the jawline, create a curved lower border to the beard. It should barely turn the corner of your jaw.

Allow the beard to grow into its full glory.

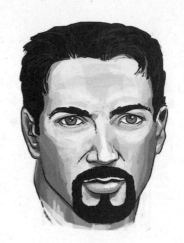

THE CIRCLE BEARD

(also known as the Door Knocker)
We've all seen it. It's the style that ruled
the '90s. Everyone from George Michael to Kurt Cobain sported the Circle
Beard—the trimmed mustache/goatee
combination that is forever inscribed in
the tomes of facial hair fashions. Like its
traditional counterpart, the circle beard
takes the style a little further by empha-
sizing a round shape. If you have a round-shaped face, however, avoid
this style and choose a version that is more square-shaped.

How to achieve this style:

Shave all hair from your cheeks and throat.

Leave a rounded beard that extends from the mustache to beneath your chin.

Trim the uppermost edge of the mustache into a curve that blends into the boundary of the beard to create a consistent round shape.

Groom the mustache and beard hairs to the desired length using scissors or an electric trimmer.

Clip the lower edge of the mustache flush with your upper lip.

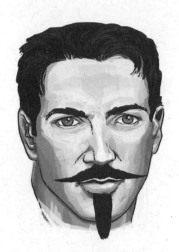

THE ROMAN T-BEARD
(also known as the Hammer-Cut or
Napoleon III Imperial)
Dating back to the early seventeenth
century, it was first referenced in 1647 in
the Beaumont and Fletcher folio of *The
Queen of Corinth*. The style combines a
straight mustache that extends from each
side of the face in straight, narrow points
with a long goatee trimmed into a point. It resembles a hammer or the
letter T, hence the nicknames. It was also a favorite of Napoleon III.

How to achieve this style:

Shave the beard clean, leaving only the chin whiskers and mustache.

Trim the beard to a long point.

The mustache should be allowed to grow to a length great enough to mold into horizontal points.

Apply a medium-hold mustache wax sparingly to both the whiskers on your chin and
mustache to hold the style's pointed look.

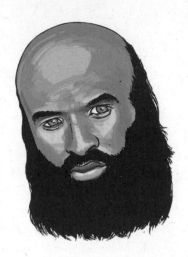

THE CATHEDRAL BEARD

This favorite style of Santa Claus, Leonardo da Vinci, and sixteenth-century men of the cloth is truly a celebration of the beard. It is accomplished by cultivating a full, bushy beard that extends down to the chest in cascades of flowing whiskers. The mustache and beard come together seamlessly and conceal the skin underneath. The style is traditionally worn square cut or rounded, but never forked or pointed.

Variations on the Cathedral Beard include the Sugarloaf Beard, which is also a long style but worn narrower at the bottom than the top, resulting in a soft point at the tip.

How to achieve this style:

This style requires several months of growth to achieve, so get started now!

Trim your cheek area to an even length, shorter than the chin and mustache whiskers.

Allow your mustache and chin whiskers to grow freely, grooming them downward into a broad curtain that extends beneath the collar.

Wash your beard everyday using face wash and rinse with a conditioner to keep it soft.

Comb your beard daily to remove any loose hairs, prevent knots, and keep it clean of leaves, twigs, crumbs, and small woodland creatures.

THE SPADE BEARD

(variations also known as the Shenandoah, *Pique Devant*, Marquisette, or Chin Curtain)

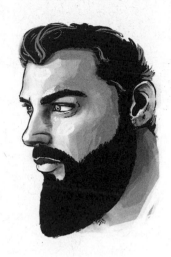

There seem to be some varying definitions of what makes a Spade Beard. Some say it includes a thick, natural mustache and others say it does not. Without a mustache, a Spade beard appears similar to a Chin Curtain style (see page 80)—one that is worn full on the cheeks and chin but remains clean-shaven above the upper lip.

In the sixteenth century, the Spade meant a long goatee with a full, Handlebar-style mustache and clean-shaven cheeks. But these days, people consider the Spade to be similar to what used to be called a *Pique Devant*, which is a natural mustache and beard that features long growth extending from the chin to create a blunt point. One might say it's similar to a Stiletto beard (see page 72) but without the pointed shape.

How to achieve this style:

Allow your beard and mustache to grow freely for several months.

The cheek line is left natural, as is the mustache.

Using scissors and a comb, trim your chin whiskers to a uniform length.

Using scissors, shape the chin and jaw whiskers to form a broad, blunt point that extends a few inches below your chin.

Apply medium-hold mustache wax sparingly (if needed).

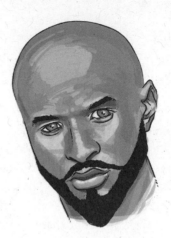

THE STILETTO BEARD

Depending on the wearer, the Stiletto Beard makes a sharp style statement that is either menacing or heroic. A pointed mustache and a beard that extends a few inches from the chin into a point add some major angles to any face. Associated with imagery of the devil, the sharp points of a Stiletto Beard look like they could be hazardous to the health of anyone who gets too close. Proceed with caution, or use a softer wax.

How to achieve this style:

Grow your beard and mustache naturally.

Once sufficient length is achieved (after about six to eight weeks of unchecked growth), apply wax to the outer areas of your mustache to create points that extend from your face, curving slightly outwards.

Using a pair of facial hair scissors, trim lower beard whiskers to a point extending a few inches below your chin.

If needed, apply a small amount of wax to the end of the point to retain its shape.

Your cheek line may be left natural, or for a more severe look, shave borders into sharp edges extending from the ears to the mustache.

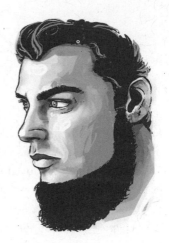

THE AMISH (DUTCH) BEARD

The Amish, a bearded Christian sect, are the followers of Jakob Ammann, who provided them with specific instructions on such practices as washing their feet and trimming their beards. Primarily members of the old order of the Amish Mennonites, they first moved from Europe to North America around 1720, with additional migrations following in the nineteenth and twentieth centuries. The Amish settled in a wide area of North America that includes Pennsylvania, Kansas, and Ontario. Known for steadfastly adhering to their traditional ways, Amish men continue to be noted for their broad-brimmed black hats, their homemade clothes with hooks and eyes but no store-bought buttons, and their characteristic beards without mustaches. In some Amish communities, such a beard also indicates that a man is married.

Although this style requires at least three months' natural growth, one can achieve a shorter version if desired.

How to achieve this style:

Shave all hair from your cheeks to the base of the smile lines, forming a curving line from your sideburns to your chin.

With scissors and a comb, trim the beard from your sideburns to the bottom of the smile lines, working down each side of your face to achieve a uniform length.

Using a safety razor, shave away the mustache and define the growth line of the beard.

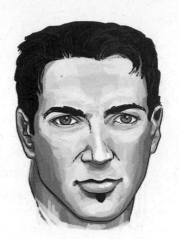

THE SOUL PATCH

(also known as a Flavor Saver or Royale)
The Soul Patch is a style staple for the
collegiate set. While it used to be considered a man's first step toward facial hair
(especially if he's follicularly challenged),
it has begun to gain support as a simple
way to experiment with facial hair without going for the whole woolly beard.

How to achieve this style:

Shave all hair from your cheeks, neck, and chin.

Shave your upper lip clean.

Leave only the hair immediately beneath the lower lip.

These whiskers can be shaped into a triangular patch, with angles reaching a point in the
center of the chin; create a solid square, shaving a straight line down from your lower lip to
the chin; or form a softer circular tuft using scissors or a razor.

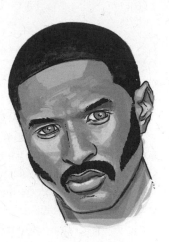

THE SHAFT BEARD

Named for the 1971 blaxploitation film, adapted from a novel by the same name that tells the story of a black private detective, John Shaft, who travels through Harlem in search of a black mobster's missing daughter. Shaft is known for his no-nonsense approach and even more no-nonsense beard, a distinctive mustache paired with sideburns trimmed high to emphasize the cheekbones.

How to achieve this style:

Trim your entire beard to a uniform length of about a quarter inch. This is best achieved using an electric trimmer.

Shave your cheeks clean, leaving the curving hairline from your sideburns to the outer tips of your mustache.

Similarly, shave under the jaw, forming a curving line stretching from each ear to the point at which the throat and lower jaw meet, just about at the Adam's apple.

Trim the uppermost mustache edge beneath your nose, defining a horizontal line.

Leaving the natural hairline intact, trim above your upper lip.

Shape the whiskers between the lower lip and chin to form a narrow stripe or Soul Patch. Can you dig it?

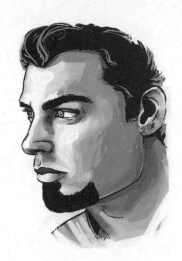

THE GOATEE

A true (if a tad ubiquitous) classic, the Goatee sets the foundation for many facial hair looks. Inspired by the charming hairs that hang from the chin of a goat, it can add length to any man's face and enhance a soft jaw. The goatee is commonly paired with a mustache.

This particular style can also be worn in a wider form, occupying more real estate beneath the chin, if desired. A wider-width goatee is an excellent choice for men with particularly pointed chins. Experiment with widths until you find one that best suits your face.

How to achieve this style:

Shave your cheeks and throat clean.

Shave your chin whiskers, leaving hair only on the region below the boundary of the mouth. This hair may be trimmed short or groomed to a longer point.

Shave below your lower lip, removing the Soul Patch whiskers.

Shave the area between the corners of your mouth and the chin, forming a sharp boundary where your chin whiskers begin.

THE ANCHOR BEARD

With nautical-inspired trends a perennial favorite on fashion runways, why not show some sailor pride in your beard? The anchor is another wonderfully descriptive name for a beard that resembles a ship's anchor. It extends from beneath the jaw to form a point directly below the chin. Hair is short at the outermost edges of the jawline and longest in the middle of the chin to create a point. A thin strip of hair connects the Soul Patch (see page 74) to the beard. With this style, the mustache is usually an angular pencil-thin or pyramidal shape.

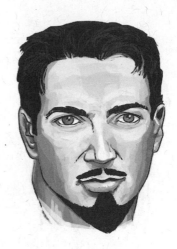

How to achieve this style:

Shave your cheeks clean.

Using your jaw line as a guide, shave away hair above the jaw bone, to outline your jaw.

Using scissors and a comb or an electric trimmer, cut the hair along your jaw line down to a quarter to half an inch in length. Start with the outermost edges of the jawline (closest to your ears) first, where hair is shortest. As you move closer to your chin, hair should get longer with the longest whiskers directly beneath the chin.

Below your lower lip, shave away the hair at the corners of your mouth that extend to the sides of your chin. Leave only the Soul Patch and the hair below it that connects to the whiskers at the center of your chin.

Allow the whiskers beneath your chin to grow for a few weeks while using a pair of scissors to carefully create the pointed shape.

Use a bit of mustache wax to create a perfect point, or wear it natural for a softer look. Ahoy, matey!

THE BALBO BEARD

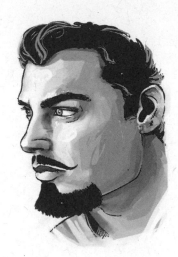

A wild facial hair cocktail, the Balbo consists of a wide Goatee (see page 52), Chinstrap (see page 82), and a Handlebar mustache (see page 76). Similar to the Goatee, the whiskers beneath the chin are cultivated into a full display, extending two inches beyond both corners of the mouth. On the neck, this beard should extend to the natural border where the chin meets the neck. A narrow strip of hair also runs from the lower lip to the chin. For a final act, the mustache is styled into a Handlebar shape with gently upturned ends. It is a style that will surely one-up your bewhiskered buddies.

How to achieve this style:

Shave your cheeks clean.

Create a lower border where your neck meets your chin and shave everything below it clean.

Cultivate the whiskers beneath your chin extending three inches from the center on both sides, shaving the rest.

Remove the hair between the corners of your lips to your chin.

Using an outliner, create a narrow, rectangular strip of hair extending from your lower lip to your chin.

Allow your mustache to grow for three to four weeks.

Once you have cultivated an ample length, create a part in the middle of the lip crease with a straight razor or outliner.

Using a medium-hold mustache wax, brush each half of your mustache outward toward the tips and curl the ends upward.

THE BRETT BEARD

This style combines the Chinstrap beard (see page 82) with the Soul Patch (see page 74). The whiskers along the jaw line are grown to create a carefully manicured line that connects with the Soul Patch. It adds a little more shape to the Chinstrap style, and the extra whiskers on the chin helps it look more pronounced. An important difference between the Brett and the Chinstrap is that the Brett does not connect with the sideburns. Instead, it follows the jawline to the ears. Because this style relies on its defined shape, daily upkeep is key.

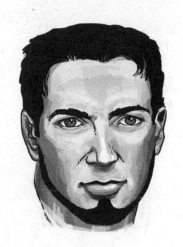

How to achieve this style:

Shave your cheeks and mustache clean.

Along the jawline, leave a strip of hair the runs from ear to ear.

Allow the hair on your chin and Soul Patch whiskers to remain intact, but shave those that connect the corner of the mouth to your chin.

Trim the beard to a uniform length of a quarter to a half inch.

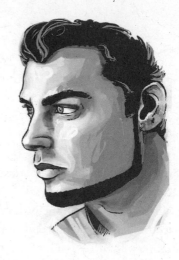

THE CHIN CURTAIN BEARD

This is a North American name for a narrow band of whiskers around the face and chin.

How to achieve this style:

Shave your cheeks clean in a slope following the sideburn line, downward to a point two inches above the jaw.

Form a curving upper beard edge that extends from your sideburn line to your chin, leaving chin whiskers intact.

Shave away your mustache and hair beneath the lower lip.

Groom the beard length and chin whiskers to a dull point, using scissors and a comb.

THE CHIN PUFF

Simply a Chinstrip (see page 83) cultivated into a long tuft that begins at the
lower lip and extends down to the chin,
the Chin Puff may even hang off the
chin if desired. This style, too, requires
fastidious upkeep to maintain the clear
borders of the strip.

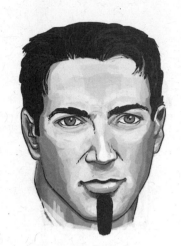

How to achieve this style:

Shave your cheeks, mustache, and neck clean.

When shaving the chin, proceed to leave a half-inch strip of hair between the lower lip and
the chin. The strip may curve under the chin if you desire.

After a few weeks of solid growth, use an outliner or straight razor to create sharp
boundaries on all four sides of the rectangular shape.

Allow your whiskers to grow to any desired length. The longer they become, the more
dramatic the puff will be—and we do love a dramatic puff!

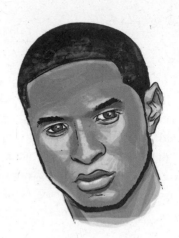

THE CHINSTRAP BEARD
(also known as the Jaw line Beard)
Not to be confused with the Chinstrip
or Landing Strip (see opposite), the
Chinstrap became a popular style in
the late twentieth and early twenty-
first century, commonly worn by young
people. The style can be described as a
thin half- to one-inch strip of hair that
begins with one sideburn, continues down to the chin, follows the jaw
line past the chin to the other side and then up the face to connect with
the opposite sideburn. It emphasizes (or creates) a strong jaw line while
minimizing the beard's appearance on the face. It also demands great
self-discipline to shape and maintain on a regular basis.

How to achieve this style:

Grow your beard for one to two weeks to create ample growth for consistent length.

Using scissors or electric trimmer, crop the beard to a quarter-inch.

Using a razor, carve a half-inch line straight down from your sideburns to the jaw line. Be
sure to keep the width consistent.

Following the jaw line, carve a half-inch line to the center of your chin on both sides of the
face, creating one continuous strip from one sideburn to the other.

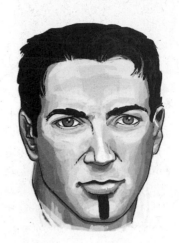

THE LANDING STRIP BEARD

(also known as The Chinstrip)
While the Chinstrip is similar in name
to the Chinstrap, that's as far as the
similarities go. This is a variation on
the Soul Patch (see page 74). Instead of
a small patch of hair growing beneath
the lower lip, it forms a strip of hair
that extends from the lip to the bottom
of the chin. Not all men can grow this
style due to some sparse growth between the Soul Patch and the chin,
but it's a great option for the follicularly blessed men with round faces.

How to achieve this style:

Shave your cheeks, mustache, and neck clean.

When shaving the chin, proceed to leave a half-inch strip of hair between the lower lip and the chin. The strip may curve under the chin if you desire.

After a few weeks of solid growth, use an outliner or straight razor to create sharp boundaries on all four sides of the rectangular shape.

Using scissors and a comb, or an electric trimmer, cut all the whiskers to a uniform length of your choosing—usually a quarter to half an inch in length.

Now stroke your Chinstrip in a thoughtful manner.

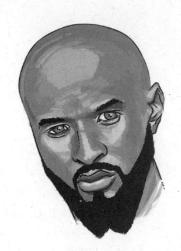

THE FRENCH FORK

The varieties of forked beards are many, but perhaps the most well-known is the French Fork for its long, thick, pointed fork design. This beard extends a few inches from the chin to the chest. The section extending from the chin is divided into two distinct sections to create a forked appearance. Each section comes to a point.

Other variations include the Swallowtail, which is reserved for beards that feature more dramatically spread sections.

How to achieve this style:

Allow your beard to grow for six to eight weeks.

Trim the whiskers on your cheeks to approximately half to three-quarters of an inch in length while leaving the hair on your chin to grow uninterrupted.

Divide the hair extending from your chin into two distinct sections and pull them apart.

Trim and brush each section into a point. Apply a bit of wax if your whiskers fail to hold the style.

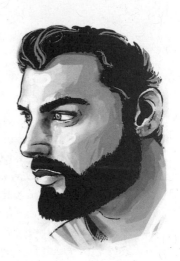

THE FULL BEARD

Perhaps the easiest style to grow, the
full beard just takes patience—and
ample whiskers. The Full Beard
is exactly that, one that covers the
mustache, cheeks, chin, and neck. It
can be worn at a variety of lengths
to various degrees of fullness—from
close-cropped to a fuller look worthy
of Jolly Old Saint Nick. Guys with
sparse whiskers or barren patches will have a difficult time cultivating
the necessary follicles to create the look. The Full Beard can also be
tailored to suit any face shape.

How to achieve this style:

Avoid shaving for three weeks to see if your beard has any patchy or sparse areas.

While continuing to grow your beard for several weeks, you may begin to add some desired
shape and trim the edges along the neck and cheeks if you so choose.

Using a comb and facial hair scissors or an electric trimmer, trim away the extra long
whiskers to create a uniform length on your cheeks.

On the neck, create a subtle border where your whiskers become visibly sparse. Leaving
these strays behind will make you look unkempt (or like a vagrant).

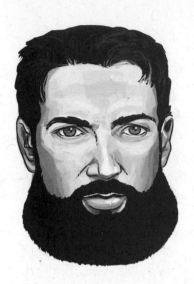

THE GARIBALDI BEARD

This beard is one hell of a style statement. Named after the nineteenth-century Italian military and political hero Giuseppe Garibaldi, this particularly full beard features a large half-circle shape extending from the jaw. Because of its round shape, guys with round faces should steer clear if they hope to balance out their facial structure.

How to achieve this style:

Allow your beard to grow unchecked for two to three months.

Comb and condition your beard a few times a week or more to keep it healthy and soft.

Using facial hair scissors, trim the whiskers on your cheeks slightly to create a uniform length, leaving the natural borders of the beard intact. Do not cut into the beard—just trim the strays.

The whiskers along your jaw line and chin should be allowed to grow longer than the rest of the beard.

After cultivating adequate length, use a pair of facial hair scissors to begin shaping the beard into a half circle beginning at one ear and proceeding to the other.

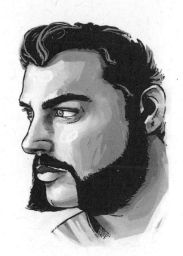

THE HULIHEE BEARD

This style is a Hawaiian beard, distinguished by its fat chops connected to a well-groomed mustache. The word is derived from the Hawaiian *hulihe'e*, meaning "turn and flee," which doesn't do this particular style much justice.

How to achieve this style:

Grow your beard for four to six weeks.

Shave your chin and the area of your neck immediately below your chin clean, leaving your mustache and cheek whiskers intact.

The uppermost border of your beard along the cheeks is left natural, but can be groomed using a razor if hair growth spreads too high or is particularly unruly. If you choose to tidy up, using a razor, create a top border by shaving a sloped line along the natural border of your beard to your mouth.

Use scissors to trim your mustache to a neat length of about half an inch.

Encourage your long chops to flare outwards by applying medium-hold wax or sculpting with a beard comb.

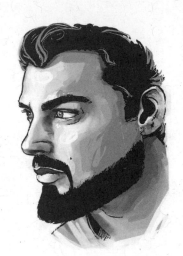

THE HOLLYWOODIAN BEARD

Don't expect to see the Hollywood-ian Beard on the red carpet anytime soon (although we do love a good comeback). This throwback style is a little piece of vintage Hollywood glamour. A variation on the boxed beard, the Hollywoodian features a full beard with cropped cheeks, a connected mustache, and a Chinstrip (see page 83).

How to achieve this style:

Allow your beard to grow for three to four weeks.

Shave the upper half of the beard on your cheeks, leaving a sloped line extending from your ear to the top of your chin. Do not connect the beard to your sideburns.

Following the natural line where your neck connects with your chin, create a lower boundary for your beard.

Leave a thin vertical line at each side of your mouth, connecting your mustache to your beard.

Using a straight razor or outliner, trim the Soul Patch into a rectangular chin strip.

Allow the beard to grow into the desired fullness. You may wish to use a pair of facial hair scissors to clip away stray hairs and create a uniform length on the cheeks.

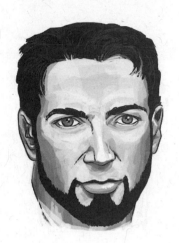

THE KLINGON

This favorite among Trekkies and sci-fi
enthusiasts earned its name from the beloved alien race in *Star Trek*. The Kling-
on beard isn't difficult for the human
race to achieve. In fact, it's as simple as
growing a full beard but shaving away the
mustache directly above the lip and leaving the whiskers between the mustache
and chin intact.

How to achieve this style:

Allow your beard to grow for four to six weeks.

Using scissors or an electric trimmer, cut the whiskers directly above your lip as short as possible.

Using a razor, remove the hair directly above your lip while leaving the whiskers that connect your chin and mustache untouched.

Create a strong border on your neck where it meets your chin and shave the rest of your neck clean.

Live long and prosper.

THE SPARROW

Even Disney films inspire facial hair designs. Johnny Depp's beard in *Pirates of the Caribbean* was almost as memorable as his performance. The Sparrow, named after Depp's character, Jack Sparrow, features a full mustache, Soul Patch (see page 74), and a Goatee (see page 76). For added drama, the Goatee includes two long braids dangling from the chin. The ornamental beads are optional.

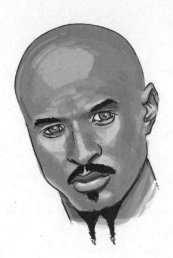

How to achieve this style:

Shave all hair from your cheeks and neck.

Leave the hair above the upper lip and beneath the lower lip and chin untouched.

The mustache should extend slightly below the corners of your mouth to create a frame around the lips.

Using an outliner or straight razor, trim the Soul Patch into a triangular shape that is wide at the top and points to the chin.

The Goatee's width should extend about one inch beyond the corners of the mouth. Use an outliner or straight razor to create the necessary borders.

Beneath your chin, the Goatee should be allowed to grow at least four to five inches in length.

Part the goatee into two strands and braid each section individually.

Add colorful beads, matey, and work on your best pirate impression.

THE VAN DYKE BEARD
(also Vandyke, VanDyke, Van Dyck)

This style was named after the seventeenth-century Flemish painter Sir Anthony Van Dyke (also spelled Van Dyck), who was known for his religious-themed paintings and regal portraits (in which many of the big-shots sported beards just like his). Typically, the style consists of a short, pointy beard and a waxed pointy mustache, without hair on the side of the face.

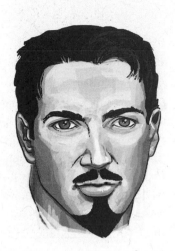

How to achieve this style:

Stop shaving for about one week. At this point, your whiskers will be shorter than necessary to achieve this style; however, you can begin shaping it while keeping the rest of your face clean-shaven.

Using a razor, shave your cheeks clean, leaving your chin whiskers and mustache intact.

As your chin beard (goatee) grows longer, carefully trim into a pointed shape using scissors and a careful technique. You don't want to trim too deeply into the beard or snip off the tip you've worked so hard to grow!

Twist the ends of your mustache into points, applying a light-weight wax to maintain the shape.

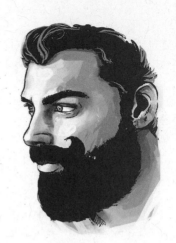

THE VERDI BEARD

Named after the Italian romantic composer Giuseppe Verdi, this specific style offers a dash of old-world romance and like a classic opera, the Verdi beard is always in fashion. The cropped style is kept relatively short and features a rounded bottom shape and a full, upturned mustache. (Men with rounder faces might want to avoid this style due to the rounded shape.)

How to achieve this style:

Allow your beard to grow untouched for three to four weeks before attempting to lay the groundwork for the shape.

Following the natural line where your neck connects with your chin, create a lower boundary for your beard.

With a pair of scissors and a comb, gently trim the whiskers on your cheeks while leaving your mustache untouched.

Using a small amount of mustache wax (if desired), curl the corners of the mustache upward.

Allow your beard to grow into the desired fullness. Using a pair of facial hair scissors, trim the lower portion of the beard into a rounded shape. Sing with confidence in the shower!

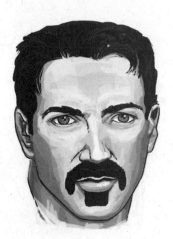

THE ZAPPA

The Zappa is an homage to musician Frank Zappa, who sported a combination mustache and Soul Patch (see page 74). The corners of the mustache should extend slightly below the corners of the mouth to create a boxy shape.

How to achieve this style:

Shave all hair from your cheeks, neck, and chin.

Leave only the hair immediately beneath your lower lip and the mustache untouched.

The mustache should extend slightly below the corners of your mouth to create a subtle frame around the lips.

Using an outliner or straight razor, trim the Soul Patch into a square or wide rectangle.

If you want to pay homage to Zappa, wear the style thick and full. Allow your whiskers to grow for a few weeks to create a fuller look.

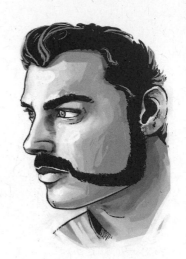

À LA SUVAROV

This style just might be the predecessor to the Chinstrap (see page 82)—but don't quote us on that. Beginning with the sideburn, it creates a strip of hair that runs down to the jawline, follows the jaw to just below the corner of the mouth, and then curves upward to connect with the mustache. It can be worn in a curved shape or a more boxy, squarish style that's great for guys with round faces. One might guess that the style was pioneered by the eighteenth-century Russian military leader Alexander Suvarov, but most images depict him looking rather clean-shaven.

How to achieve this style:

Allow your beard to grow for four to six weeks.

Shave your chin and neck clean.

Allow your mustache to grow slightly below the corners of your mouth.

Shave your right sideburn into a J-like shape that grows straight down to the chin, then curves up to connect with your mustache.

Repeat the last step on the left side of your face so it is a mirror image of the other.

Keep the style relatively short—about a quarter to half an inch in length. Your mustache may be worn slightly longer for a fuller appearance.

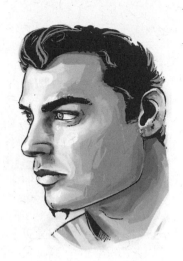

EL INSECTO
(also known as the Mighty)
El Insecto is not a common style, but deserves mention. This particular look features two small curled points extending from the chin and resembles the facial features of an insect. This style is probably best reserved for Halloween, but if you can pull it off with swagger, we wish you luck.

How to achieve this style:

Shave your cheeks, mustache and neck, leaving just two patches at the bottom of the corners of your chin.

Cultivate the whiskers to grow at least an inch in length.

Use a tiny amount of mustache wax to mold them into curled, insect-like tendrils.

Proceed to scare your dog and the neighborhood kids.

The Step-by-Step Style Guide to Sideburns

SIDEBURNS (STANDARD ISSUE)

Don't underestimate the seductive power of sideburns. Too often they are overlooked as a great style option.

Sported by men throughout history from Ralph Waldo Emerson to Elvis Presley, sideburns can change the appearance of your face. Men with round-shaped faces can benefit greatly from the slimming effect provided by the vertical lines of sideburns. The standard issue styles are neatly shaped vertical lines that maintain a constant width from top to bottom. They can be worn at any length and by men with just about any face shape. Guys with longer faces should wear their sideburns shorter (if they wear them at all) to minimize the length and narrowness of the face (the vertical line of 'burns doesn't do them any favors).

There are four common lengths of standard-issue sideburns:

1. Short sideburns grow just half- to one inch below the top of the ear.
2. Medium sideburns grow to the length of the middle of the ear.
3. Long sideburns grow to the bottom of the ear lobe.
4. Extra-long sideburns grow between the bottom of the earlobe and the jaw line.

How to achieve this style:

Shave as usual, leaving the sideburns untouched.

After one to two weeks, you can begin to determine the shape of your sideburns. Using a razor, create a lower border by shaving a clear horizontal line where you want your sideburn to end. Shave all the hair below that line.

If you are growing medium to extra-long sideburns, use your razor to create strong vertical borders from the top to bottom. The sideburns should maintain the same width.

Use scissors and a comb or an electric trimmer to keep sideburn whiskers at a uniform length.

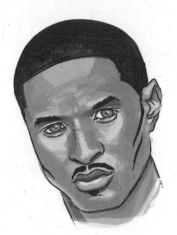

TAPERED

Tapered sideburns begin at their normal width and as they descend, they become a pointed shape. Grown similarly to standard issue sideburns, this style requires a little fastidious grooming and razor precision to maintain the edgy look.

How to achieve this style:

Shave as usual while leaving your sideburns untouched for one to two weeks.

Using a razor, create a vertical line that extends from the top of the sideburn and angles toward the middle.

Repeat the last step with the other side of the sideburn to create a point.

Use an electric trimmer or scissors, and comb to create a uniform hair length.

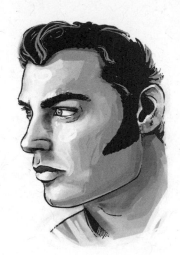

FLARED

Flared sideburns begin above the ear at about three-quarters to one inch in width and grow wider as they descend toward the jaw line. This particular style works well for men who wish to slim their face shapes and highlight their cheekbones.

Pairing flared sideburns with a Horseshoe mustache (see page 57) creates a classic style called the Winnfield.

How to achieve this style:

Grow your beard for one to two weeks.

As your sideburns become more visible, create a lower border at your desired length by shaving a defined, horizontal line at the bottom. This line should be somewhere between your ear lobes and your chin to achieve the flared appearance.

Shave your neck, chin, and mustache clean.

If you prefer a blocked shape, shave an angled line from the top of the sideburn to the wider bottom edge.

If you prefer a swooping curved design, use a razor to create a sloping line from your ear to the tip of your sideburn that follows the natural upper border of your beard.

MUTTON CHOPS

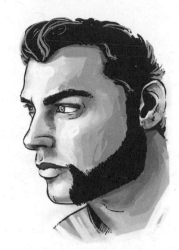

(also known as Dundrearies)
Mutton Chops earned their name
because their shape resembles
a big slab of lamb on your face.
While that might not sound
entirely appetizing, they remain
a popular and dramatic sideburn
style. They follow the natural
growth of the beard and stop
before meeting the mouth. Some
people—particularly men with rounder
faces—can benefit from a more square style. Men with pointed chins
should avoid this look because it will highlight the area.

How to achieve this style:

Grow your beard for four to six weeks.

Shave your neck, chin, and mustache clean.

Using a razor, create a top border by shaving a sloped line along the natural border of your beard to your mouth.

Shave a half- to one-inch vertical strip on both sides of your mouth to separate your mustache and mutton chops.

Create a lower border by shaving a defined line along your jaw line.

Allow your new chops to grow to the desired length. The bushier, the better! Start smoking a pipe and guffaw at every opportunity.

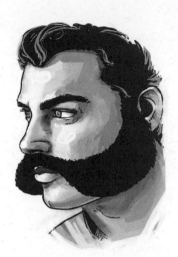

BURNSIDES
(also known as Friendly Mutton Chops)
Named after American Civil War Brigadier General Ambrose Burnside, this particular style is also known as Friendly Mutton Chops. Both sideburns extend to the jaw line and create a mutton-chop-like shape. They then angle upward to connect with the mustache to highlight the chin. A style like this takes six to eight weeks to achieve, but it's possible to build the foundations for the shape much earlier.

How to achieve this style:

Shave your chin and neck clean, leaving the mustache intact.

Allow your sideburns to grow down to your jaw and extend halfway to your chin.

Shave the top edge of your cheeks, leaving the sideburns and a one-and-a-half–inch strip of hair intact.

The sideburns should then connect with the mustache at a forty-five-degree angle to create a triangular shape.

Trim the top of the mustache to create a defined line and a Chevron-like shape.

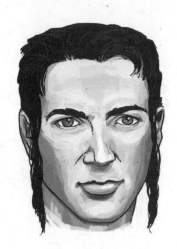

PEYOT
(also spelled *Peya, Peyot, Payos, Peyes, Pe'ahs,* and known also as Sidelocks)
The long and curled Sidelocks worn by Orthodox sects of the Jewish faith deserve mention. The Torah says, "You shall not round the corners of your heads, neither shall you mar the corners of your beard" (Lev. 19:27). *Peyot,* meaning corners, is believed to refer to the sideburns, so many leave them untrimmed. Cutting them was considered a sin or heathen practice. If they aren't worn in their full ringleted glory, they are often tucked behind the ears.

Peyot take many months to cultivate—especially if you wish to rock the curls—so be patient. Interestingly, non-Jewish college kids have recently adopted this style on campuses all over the place.

How to achieve this style:

Shave your beard, mustache, and chin clean.

Some believe you should not shave any part of your sideburns from the ear down to a level that is even with the tip of the nose. Below the nose is fair game.

Wait for months until adequate growth is achieved.

If your sideburns are not naturally curly, you might consider applying some light-hold gel to them and wrapping them around a pen or pencil.

Other Facial Hair Styles

STUBBLE

A favorite of the red carpet Hollywood set, stubble adds an air of bad boy rebellion. But it can also be a difficult style to manage. Its short crop requires near-daily maintenance to achieve that "I-just-woke-up" look. Stubble is a great way to slim the lower half of the face and to highlight your cheekbones. Men with particularly square or angular faces can further emphasize their face shapes with this particular style, but should use caution if they don't want to look like a back alley heroin addict.

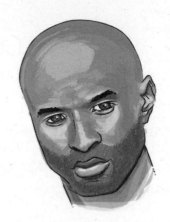

How to achieve this style:

Avoid the razor for one to two days.

Create a lower border by shaving along the line where your chin meets your neck and remove all hair below it. (There's no excuse for an unkempt neck.)

Using an electric trimmer, clip your whiskers to a uniform length.

Along the edges of your beard, choose a setting that is one step shorter than before. This will blend the edges to create a more natural look.

FREESTYLE

Freestyle means using your creativity to brave uncharted territory! Go wherever your imagination takes you. Mix and match wild, bushy sideburns with a neat and tidy Pencil-thin mustache, or accent your Cathedral beard with spokes like a carriage wheel. The permutations and possibilities are endless. Go forth bravely in your hirsute pursuit!

CHAPTER FOUR

MAINTENANCE

Washing, Combing, Trimming, Waxing, Snipping, Clipping, Dyeing

Washing a Beard

Do not assume that wearing a beard is a maintenance-free ride. Facial hair can get whiffy, food-filled, and may become a refuge for small living creatures if you're not careful. Beards should be washed regularly, as frequently as you wash your hair—so why not do both when you shower? If they are mild, the same products used on your scalp hair may be used to wash and condition your beard. (Some wonderful beard rinses and conditioners are also readily available; see Resources.)

If you get dandruff in your beard (yes, this can happen), using your regular dandruff shampoo in a diluted form may help. Use a small amount of shampoo or beard wash and massage it into your beard, working up a good lather. Massaging your skin and hair will make you feel pampered and will also loosen debris, skin flakes, and oil and tone up your skin. Rinse the suds off thoroughly and make sure there is no soap residue left on your beard, as this can lead to itching, flaking, clumping, and matting (as with a wet dog).

Use a small amount of hair conditioner or beard conditioner as this will enhance softness and shine (although it's unlikely to produce a marked change in the texture of your hair). Pat your beard dry with a towel. Blow-drying will irritate and dry your skin, so avoid it.

Once your beard is completely dry, you can comb it in the direction of growth with a wide-toothed comb. You can find special beard combs in the grooming aisle of your drugstore. Don't comb your hair when it's wet as this will stretch and pull your beard. After you've worked out the tangles with a comb, you may want to use a good quality beard brush with firm bristles as your final step.

Stand back and admire!

Perfect Trimming and Clipping of Beards

You basically have two options: you can use scissors or pick up an electric shaver (the cordless, rechargeable clippers are the best). If you want to go with scissors, pick up a pair of barber's shears, which are long and narrow and allow you to trim hard-to-reach areas. You also want a pair of blunt, short scissors for clipping around the ears and nostrils without gashing yourself. Grab a long, thin, narrow comb and draw out the hair that you wish to trim away. Doing this will prevent you from over-clipping and producing slow-to-grow bald spots.

Before you start trimming, make sure your beard is dry (wet hair seems longer but then springs shorter once it's dry). Use the comb to isolate the length of hair to be trimmed away. Work your way down the length of one side of your face from ear to chin, then do the same on the other side, comparing frequently to make sure the results are even.

The Electric Shaver Method

Multiple snazzy high-tech beard clippers have hit the market as manufacturers realized that facial hair is here to stay, and if you can't beat 'em (those non-shavers), join 'em. Cordless rechargeable models are the easiest to use, and some are even designed to be used in the shower.

Read the product instructions closely, but be aware that all clippers have closeness settings or various guard-comb attachments that allow you to select a specific length. Always start longer and then proceed to shorter as you won't be able to reverse excessive trimming.

Comb your dry beard in the direction of growth to work out tangles and remove stray hairs. Proceed systematically as described for the scissors method above. Begin with the upper boundary above your jaw, shaping the edge from your chin to your ears. Trim away from the hairline to avoid cutting too deeply into the body of the beard itself. Next, trim the underside from the center of the chin to below each earlobe.

For clipping the beard line, remove attachments and hold the clipper vertically with blades facing you. Be gentle and go slow! Select the comb attachment or setting that corresponds to your desired beard length and pass the shaver over the body of your beard, trimming and tapering its length and defining the edges and sideburns. The goal is uniformity. Many men like to start at the sideburn area and trim downward toward the chin. Others start at one side of the face and then compare constantly with the other for balance.

Always keep your trimmer clean as per manufacturer's instructions.

Trimming and Clipping Your Mustache

If you are going to use scissors, moisten your mustache hair and comb it straight down over your lips. Don't force it to lie completely flat as it will return to its natural growth direction when dry, and you may have discovered that you trimmed it too short. Using narrow, pointed scissors, trim outward from the center of your lip to each corner using a comb to gauge how much to trim away. Hold the scissors at a diagonal as this will give you greater control and also ensure that the line you trim is straight.

If you want a pencil-thin style or a very straight lower edge, use a clipper as directed below. Once your stache is tidy and shapely, you can use the scissors to clip away any stray, long, or unkempt hairs. Consider using mustache wax, especially for longer mustaches (see page 106).

The Electric Shaving Method

If you're going electric, make sure that your mustache hair is dry before you start. Comb it straight downward over your lips. Comb away from the mustache hairline. Define the upper edge below the nostrils. If you are going to wear your mustache with a beard, use your blending comb attachment. Make sure everything looks even. If you have only a mustache, taper it as desired using a comb attachment and working your way from the center to the corners of your mouth. You may also want to blend the mustache downward from its upper edge of growth to the rim of your upper lip, reducing the density of growth through its mid-portion. Find the lower edge using the comb and the electric shaver, taking care to trim gradually and to avoid a slip of the hand.

Sideburn Clipping

For trimming sideburns, comb them into place. Use the appropriate length guard or clipper setting. Hold the clipper vertically and trim downward. Stare at the mirror head-on so that you can compare the sideburn lengths right to left and keep things even. From time to time, let your barber do the clipping and tidying for you. He can also give you feedback on how good your home-based attempts really are.

How to Use Mustache Wax

Lots of stache wax products are available (see Resources). Buying them will make you feel like you're part of an exclusive club, one to which Salvador Dali, Hercule Poirot, and Snidely Whiplash proudly belonged. Take a smidgen—and we mean a smidgen—and

Three Old-Style Objects for Serious Mustache Wearers

• a **mustache curler** for a saucy flip

• a **mustache cup** that has a special rim that allows you to drink without getting messy

• a **snood**, which is essentially a mustache bra that you wear at night to keep things in place (Hercule Poirot was known to wear one)

rub it between your thumb and index finger. Make sure your stache is dry, and apply sparingly with one finger.

You can cover the whole mustache for an overall tidy look or just twirl the points repeatedly between your thumb and forefinger (you may wish to laugh in a sinister way as you do so).

To achieve upturning points, twirl with a technique much the same as snapping your fingers. Keep in mind that most of the products available will slightly darken the color of your facial hair. Keep some wax in your desk or briefcase and reapply as required to maintain your style. Now go find a barbershop quartet to sing with.

Dyeing a Beard

Halloween aside, why would a man want to dye his beard?

The number one reason is that his facial hair has gone gray, white, or splotchy (but not in a silver-fox attractive way). He's looking older and wants his beard to match what's left on his head (this may be helped along with some color as well). On the other hand, some men actually embrace the contrast and want, say, a deep black beard to offset their blond hair. A few brave souls will even experiment with red, orange, or blue dyes (as did the ancient Gauls).

Here's how to get the job done:

Go to your drugstore and pick out a facial hair dyeing kit (like Just for Men). Don't even think about using hair dye on your face—the chemicals are much harsher and will damage your skin. By the same token, do not use beard dye on your eyebrows or lashes unless you want to go blind (see "A Word on Eyebrows," page 108). Choose a beard shade lighter than what you have in mind; you can always go darker, but you can't go lighter. You may want to try a wash-out, ultra-temporary product before committing to a dye-job. But if you're planning on sweating or getting particularly close to someone, the added color could rub off on clothes, bed sheets, or others. Ask your barber or hairstylist for an opinion on what shade will look best.

Do a skin-patch test as recommended in the kit instructions. You'll have to wait forty-eight hours to rule out an allergic response or rash, but it's well worth it. You don't want a face full of oozing scabs.

Wash and dry your beard before using the dye. Follow the product mixing instructions closely, and be sure to wear latex gloves. Brush the product gently up and down into your beard until all the hair is covered, but don't rub it in. Set a timer to go off (usually in five minutes). Most kits come with the colorant and developer, gloves, a mixing tray, and a small applicator brush.

Rinse off the product with warm water and don't get it into your eyes. Use a gentle shampoo made for colored hair whenever you wash your beard.

Repeat as necessary once the color fades (unless your mate vetoes the idea).

Tip: If you have white or gray in your stubble and don't want to use dye, pick up some women's eyeshadow that matches or approximates your beard's normal color and rub on a light layer every morning. This works especially well for blond guys with light beards, since light blond beard dyes may be difficult to find, yet gold eyeshadow abounds! Don't be shy—head to your drugstore cosmetics counter. Never apologize. Never explain. Just hand over some dough.

A Word on Eyebrows

Just say *no* to girly shapes, over-plucking, and obvious dye jobs. If you have a unibrow, you may pluck above your nasal bridge until there is clearance and you have two eyebrows. Otherwise, get an esthetician who works with men (or your hairdresser) to tidy them up whenever you get your hair cut.

How to Apply Fake Facial Hair

Maybe you're chicken and can't commit to growing fuzz for any length of time. Maybe it's Halloween, or you need to go somewhere incognito. You can don fake fur to change your look (see Resources for suppliers, and check out youtube for how-to videos). Kits generally come with hair, glue, and instructions, but here are some generic pointers to get you started:

- Pick a color that is one or more shades lighter than the hair on your head. Give it a gentle combing and snip off loose hairs with scissors.

- For false mustaches, trim away any excess netting from the backing of the mustache, but take care not to trim too close to the hairline. Hold the mustache against your lip and trace its outline with a light eyebrow pencil. Apply a light, even coat of spirit gum to this area of the skin. If you're messy and the goop lands on your cheek, it's easily removed with rubbing alcohol or the aptly named "spirit gum remover" that often comes in the kit. Center the stache above your lip and press it on with your finger, leaving approximately an eighth of an inch between the base of the stache and the margin of your upper lip. Applying direct, even pressure along the length of the mustache will ensure that it doesn't go flying or land in your martini. Let the thing dry and resist the temptation to touch and check it. You may have to do a final tidy-up by trimming loose hairs, but go slow or there will be nothing left.

- For goatees, trim the product backing carefully. The goatee should be centered on your chin, beginning half an inch beneath your lower lip with a point extending to each corner of your mouth. Trace the outline of your goatee and apply spirit gum. Use gentle pressure to ensure that it stays on securely, and then trim as required.

- For fuller beards, ensure that the upper points are covered by or blended into your natural sideburns or hairline.

- If you're going Elvis, sideburns should blend into your natural hair. Make sure that your chops are centered evenly and that their ends reach an equal length (unless you're aiming for a Picasso-like, postmodern effect). Finally, think twice about being intimate with a new partner as the rigors of kissing sometimes dislodges false fuzz to humiliating effect.

Facial Hair for Charity: Grow a Fortune for Your Favorite Cause!

Numerous athletes, actors, and lots of us mere mortals have either sprouted facial hair or shaved it all off to raise money for causes related to cancer, children's illnesses, the homeless, hospices, and men's health issues.

The most popular and international of the lot is the Movember movement (*movember.com*) where each November, men worldwide are invited to grow a mustache to raise funds and awareness regarding prostate cancer and other men's health issues. Fun events, prizes, and contests are organized.

If you're thinking of signing on to another facial hair charitable event in your city for other causes, do your homework; make sure that the charity has a registration number and is legitimate, and then get growing or exfoliating for a good cause!

CHAPTER FIVE

SAYING GOODBYE

Shaving and Other Forms of (Temporary) Eradication

Has your woolly beard, cop stache, or goatee run its course, fallen out of fashion, or become an unbearable burden in the bathroom? It might be time for a change. Whether you want to switch up your style or clear-cut your whiskers entirely, numerous implements for hair removal are available to get the job done quickly—and painlessly.

How to Get Rid of a Beard

First of all, reflect carefully on your decision. Divorces have resulted from abrupt facial hair changes. (Even worse, others may not even notice.) Some men go into acute mourning.

To fully embrace the ritual, you may want to have your barber perform the task with hot towels, ample foam, and a straight razor. Select a suitable funeral march CD to play during this procedure. And if you are going to do this at home, close the bathroom door so that your sobs cannot be heard throughout the rest of the house. (Just kidding.)

If you have an electric razor, use it to trim away as much dry hair as you can first. Shaving during or immediately following a hot shower can reduce skin irritation and make the shaving process more comfortable. Your skin will be extra sensitive, having been spared the blade for so long, so use mild products with lots of moisturizer in them and a new, clean, sharp blade to reduce nicks, cuts, and skin abrasions.

Scrub your face gently with warm water, then apply a thick lather of foam, using your fingertips or a good quality shaving brush. Start with smoother facial regions and then progress to areas of coarser, denser growth, as these may require a longer soak before they are supple enough to shave. For an even closer shave, make a second pass against the lie of the hair (growth direction) once the initial shave is complete.

Be prepared for a shock if you haven't seen your bare face for a while. Then plan your next move.

Why, When, and How We Shave

It's all about ritual. In today's world there are few enduring ceremonies that continue to engage men no matter what society they live in. Even now, boys watch their fathers, grandfathers, and older brothers shave (or trim) and long for the day when they can enter manhood and start shaving themselves. Although really an aesthetic act of self-care, shaving is seen as an ultra-masculine pursuit. This is confirmed in the media by advertising that shows athletes and other macho men using "cutting edge" futuristic technology. Once you sprout facial hair as an adolescent, you've joined a testosterone-fuelled club, and once you start shaving it off, membership is guaranteed.

Every time a pimply youth shaves for the first time and looks in the mirror, he doesn't see peach fuzz; he sees a man. Each time he shaves, his masculinity is reaffirmed. Even if he only clips, snips, and trims, he's still in control.

Over the last hundred years, men have been convinced that a smooth face is masculine, athletic, upwardly mobile, classy, successful, and business-like. (Think Don Draper in *Mad Men*: the closeness of his shave entices potential mates and becomes part of his competitive edge in the corporate jungle.)

Advertisers and producers of shaving products know how important the daily ritual is to us, and they have tapped right in to make sure we keep doing it.

THE CLEAN-SHAVE MANIFESTO

We live by the blade as did our forebears through a ritual handed down from father to son.

The sacred act of shaving marks entry into manhood.

Clean-shavenness is next to godliness.

No blade too sharp; no shave too clean.

Shaving is a form of meditation.

A man recreates himself every morning with the art of shaving and thereby reveals his true face to the world.

A shaved face invites touch.

Our gear and motto: Strop, Mug, Brush, Blade.

Five Clean-Shaven Icons

- Don Draper of *Mad Men* (actor Jon Hamm)
- John F. Kennedy
- Robert Redford
- Tom Cruise
- Julio Iglesias

Shaving

When it comes to going from hair to bare, there's no greater tool than the razor. The tried-and-true weapon of mass whisker destruction has faithfully served countless generations—and it keeps getting better with each new model. But knowing which kind of razor to use and how to wield it can mean the difference between a smooth, hairless visage and looking like you wrestled with a cheese grater. The perennial questions still exist: Should I use an electric or manual razor? Is wet or dry shaving better? What's the deal with vibrating razors?

Wet vs. Dry Shaving

Shaving methods come down to a basic choice: wet or dry.

Most men know wet shaving as part of their morning ritual performed in the shower or at a bathroom sink with a bottle of shave gel, a blade, and copious amounts of water.

Dry shaving, on the other hand, is performed without water or any form of moisture. Dry shaving can be performed with many gadgets—manual and electric alike—but it's mostly associated with electric shavers and hair trimmers.

Dry shaving is useful if you've grown a beard or mustache for weeks, months, or decades. A razor will choke with long hairs if you don't first cut them short with a trimmer. Trying to shave through a thicket of long whiskers makes the regular ritual more painful and time consuming. To avoid a clog, break out a beard trimmer or hair clipper to trim the whiskers as short as possible (use a short blade guard or no guard at all, if you can do so without cutting yourself). It's easiest to trim hair when dry because it will stand up and reach the motorized teeth. When whiskers are wet, they lie flat against the skin and the trimmer won't provide a close and even trim.

Some brave men with particularly resilient skin can get away with using a manual razor on dry hair and skin, but it's not a recommended method of eradicating facial fuzz. Dragging a blade (especially a multi-blade cartridge razor) across dry skin and hair can feel like cruel and unusual punishment because whiskers are as strong as copper wire of the same thickness. Without softening the hair first, using heat and warm water, you'll feel the tug on each and every whisker as the blades pass. On the other cheek, guys with soft, thin, peach fuzz-like hair can survive a waterless shave with ease.

Moisture from warm water and a quality shaving gel or cream softens the beard and skin and reduces friction between the razor and skin, making the entire chore a much more comfortable (read: less razor burn and fewer ingrown hairs and nicks) experience. That's why most dermatologists recommend shaving in the shower or immediately after. It is also the reason a barber drapes warm, wet towels on your face before using a cutthroat straight razor.

Manual vs. Electric Razors

If you're buying a new razor, you face the dilemma of choosing a manual or electric model. A manual razor uses a single or multiple (count 'em— we're up to five!) blades that remove hair as your drag it across your face, neck, or other area of you body that contains an outcropping of unwanted hair. Manual razors include straight-edge, double-edged safety blades (preferred by grandfathers everywhere), and the multi-blade models that populate drugstore shelves (e.g., Gillette Fusion, Gillette Mach 3, Schick Quattro). Even though some manual razors now contain added bells and whistles (such as micro-pulses or vibrations), they remain in the manual razor category because they still only slice the hair when dragged across your face.

Most shaving experts agree that a manual, multi-blade razor provides the closest shave possible due to what's known as the hysteresis effect, which means the blades work together to draw whiskers out from the skin before cutting them. (Nothing to do with hysteria, unless you're addicted to buying every new shaving gadget that comes out.) The hysteresis effect results in slicing whiskers below the skin's surface.

So far, no electric razor has been able to duplicate the closeness of a manual razor—despite the manufacturers' best efforts and advertisements. Instead, electric razors provide convenience. Without the entire production of softening your beard and skin with warm water, applying gels, and rinsing a clogged blade cartridge every other stroke, an electric razor allows you to shave on the go without the need for water or the rest of the accoutrements of manual implements (though some electric shavers now require the use of a shave gel and water). It's no surprise that serious commuters put their electric blades to good use while sitting in bumper-to-bumper traffic on their way to the office.

The reason that electric shavers get away with such an effacement of age-old barbershop traditions is because the razors don't shave as close, so there's less friction between blade and skin—which results in less irritation. And the blades inside the gadget tend to move at a frenzied weed-whacker's speed, so your thick beard doesn't stand a chance. Because electric razors don't cut as closely as manual models, guys with dark beards or the five o'clock shadow-prone may find that they have to shave more than once a day to keep a clean-cut look when going the electric route.

Good Vibes or No Vibes?
Vibrations and micro-pulses are among the latest widespread features in manual and electric razors. What's all the fuss about? While the idea of any vibrating blade near your face might sound a bit frightening, the feature does offer some benefits. According to manufacturers, the added

vibes reduce friction between the skin and blade, making the experience more comfortable. It has been suggested that the vibrations also serve as a gentle anesthetic, distracting your nerves from shaving—a welcome relief for people with particularly coarse whiskers—and that the vibes cause whiskers to lift up and away from the skin for easier cutting. Some of these claims have been tested, some challenged, and some dismissed. Let's just say, there might have been some exaggeratin' goin' on.

Vibrating razors are not actually a new innovation. Some razors, like the Stahly Live Blade, date back to the 1960s (there are probably some earlier models as well) and featured double-edged safety blades with a wind-up vibration feature. Using a blade with micro-pulses, sonic technology, or vibrations remains a matter of personal preference (and they may be a bit more fun). Chances are that you'll receive a quality shave with or without the extra vibes.

Waxing, Epilators, Electrolysis, and Laser Hair Removal: Just for the Gals?

There are lots of ways to remove hair, but when it comes to facial hair removal, some should definitely be avoided by men and left to women.

Waxing: While ripping hair out of your body using hot wax and cloth strips works well for eradicating back hair or getting your torso ready for swimsuit season, keep the wax away from your beard! If you think waxing your back or chest hurts, then waxing your beard should be considered a brutal interrogation technique. The amount of pain from waxing is directly related to the thickness of the hair being ripped out of your skin. The thicker and more coarse the hair, the more its removal will hurt. Whiskers generally measure thicker than the hair on your chest, back, or legs. Only pubic hair comes close. Not only can waxing your beard pass as a form of torture, the act can cause trauma to the skin, resulting in irritated follicles and infections.

Epilators: Epilators yank out hair like a motorized gang of angry tweezers.

And for the same reason that you wouldn't want to wax your face, you should avoid these gadgets as well. Let women use them on their legs and underarms. (They probably have better pain tolerance than we do, anyway.) Your face will thank you.

Electrolysis and laser hair removal: Do you dream of eradicating your facial hair entirely so you won't have to shave again? Many men share that fantasy; however, think twice before you order up some electrolysis or laser hair removal. While zapping hair with electricity or lasers (including intense pulsed light) can halt beard growth for years at a time (or even permanently), the result is a feminized appearance. Some facial hair, even when you're otherwise clean-shaven, creates a masculine appearance. You do the math.

Ask the Expert: Shorty Maniace
Christopher "Shorty" Maniace wields a cut-throat razor with Zorro-like precision. As the head barber and manager of F.S.C. Barber in Manhattan's Lower East Side, he cuts, trims, and shaves a veritable who's who of the downtown crowd. Shorty has also worked with acclaimed men's grooming line Sharps to develop shaving products, appeared on VH1 as a style consultant, and earned the esteemed title of best Rock 'n' Roll Barber in New York City.

Q. What should every man have in his shaving kit?

A. Every man should have a blade, safety razor or cartridge, scissors, comb, a shaving brush, styptic powder, and alum stick. If he's going to be grooming tight lines, like the edges of a goatee, he should invest in a straight blade. A pre-shave oil is also important. Look for a formula that is super thin. If it feels thicker than olive oil, chances are it will clog your pores and cause ingrown hairs and irritation. If it's too sticky, it can also clog your razor. I like Musgo Real, which is almost like water. I prefer pre-shave creams that are designed to be rinsed off easily without leaving oily residue. Sharps, Proraso, and American Crew all make good ones.

Q. What kind of mustache wax do you recommend?

A. The Clubman seems to be what everybody goes for, but Skippy's Mustache Wax out of Norway is great. I've seen rave reviews about it. The thicker of our pomades, called Hawleywood's Layrite, also works well as a mustache wax. Some of the guys who do the beard competitions buy it by the ton.

Q. What is the proper way to use mustache wax?

A. Rub a little between your fingers to heat it up. This softens it and makes it easier to spread. Run it through your mustache or beard to weigh down the stray hairs that want to pop up. Or if you want to make it twirl or curl on the ends, work it into that shape and then let it cool.

Q. How do you recommend that guys treat and prevent razor burn?

A. Use proper shaving products and water that's as hot as possible when you shave. I recommend shaving in the direction of the growth first, then against the growth—if your skin isn't too sensitive. Using a pre-shave oil or cream also offers great protection against razor burn.

When shaving, use light, gentle strokes. Don't apply too much pressure to the razor and don't move too quickly. Don't rush it. Take your time. Your skin will thank you. Be with yourself for a moment in the mirror. Enjoy it—there's something soothing about shaving each morning. Once you're done shaving, use an aftershave balm that doesn't contain alcohol in order to comfort the skin. And definitely use a moisturizer.

Q. What's your cure for razor bumps?

A. There are several techniques for preventing razor bumps, which are ingrown hairs. I recommend taking a clean, dry terry washcloth and gently brushing it over the shaved area against the growth of facial hair. That will help to pull hair out and away from the face like Velcro, so it doesn't want to grow back in and cause trouble. At the end of my morning shave, I use an ice cube on my face to close the pores, and that helps prevent razor bumps, too.

How to Build a Shaving Kit

A shaving kit reveals a lot about the man who carries it. A man's kit is sacred. It contains the items a guy can't live without whether he's at home or traveling. No matter where your work or play might take you, these are the things every bearded (or mustachioed) gentleman should know before hitting the drugstore or the tarmac. From choosing the right equipment to the perfect potions and lotions, we've got you covered. Consider this your cheat sheet to Gadgets and Goopology 101.

Gadgets
Multi-blade razor

Unless you're a pro at wielding a straight-edge, reach for your favorite multi-blade razor. Ranging from two to five blades, it comes in a number of models to pick from and depends on your personal preference. Steer clear of disposable razors—they don't adjust to the facial contours as well and cause more nicks and cuts. Also, stay away from single-blade (or dollar-store) models, which don't cut as close.

Slant/point tweezers

The combination tweezer includes both a slanted and pointed end so you can grab multiple hairs with the slant or remove ingrown hairs with the pointed end. It's the perfect all-around grooming tool.

Facial hair scissors

A small but sharp pair of straight scissors allows you to work more confidently and trim more accurately than a larger pair. This means you're less likely to snip an ear or nose while trimming your mustache and beard.

Electric trimmer

If you need to give your beard or mustache a quick trim or decide it's time to remove your facial hair all together, you'll need an electric trimmer. Choose one that includes various sizes of blade guards so you can control the length.

Comb

More than just a tool to style your hair, a quality comb is vital to your facial hair trimming needs. A mustache comb has narrow teeth and is smaller in size than your usual hair comb, which makes it easier to wield around your mustache. Beard combs are also available and typically have wider teeth to help tame facial frizz. Combing your beard or mustache is great for removing old scraggly whiskers, styling your facial hair into ornate shapes, and for looking well-groomed.

Nose/ear hair scissors

While the removal of nose and ear hair isn't exactly part of shaving, these two types of facial hair deserve mention in the must-eradicate category. We recommend removing excess hair from your nose and ears as often as possible, with these specially designed blunt-tipped scissors.

Goopology
Moisturizer

The right moisturizer can help your skin recover after shaving, protect it from the elements, and keep it looking healthy. A good moisturizer doesn't have to cost a bundle either. For best results, pick up a formula that contains sunscreens that fight both UVA and UVB rays. We'll let you in on a secret: almost all alcohol-free aftershaves are moisturizers in disguise. If you're pressed for space in your luggage, leave the aftershave at home and just pack a quality, oil-free moisturizer.

Pre-shave oil

Add a little more slip to your shave with a pre-shave oil. Applied before the shaving cream, it helps soften the skin and beard, reducing friction between the blade and your face, which, in turn, greatly reduces irritation, ingrown hairs, nicks, and more. A must-have for anyone with sensitive skin. While you might be thinking that using an oil on your skin goes against just about every skin care rule, you can rest easy knowing that shaving oils won't clog your pores or cause breakouts.

Shaving cream, soap, or gel

Toss that old-school aerosol can! Shaving foam is generally not recommended. Despite its fluffy texture, it fails to provide enough skin-protecting lubricant and moisture to your skin before shaving. Gel formulas are a step up from classic foam, and companies are adding more moisturizing ingredients, but some gels are still loaded with chemical propellants, artificial colors, and heavy fragrances that can irritate skin. If you prefer a gel, find one that works with your skin instead of against it. Or toss in a cream, gel, or a shaving soap with a high fat content. Which you choose is a matter of personal preference depending on texture, moisture, and scent. Experiment until you find the one that works best for your skin.

Alum block

A crystal-like mineral stone made of alum and potassium, this is nature's own coagulant and antiseptic. That means it stops nicks from bleeding and prevents infections. Just wet the stone with water and rub it over your freshly shaved skin. You might feel a slight sting while using the block, but it's much better than leaving the house with bits of tissue stuck to your face. (However, guys with dry or sensitive skin might find the block too drying or irritating due to its astringent properties.)

Styptic pencil

Made of the same natural coagulant as an alum block, but in a pencil form. It is great for stopping bleeding when you nick or cut yourself with a razor, but its pencil shape makes using it all over your face more time-consuming.

Aftershave

Toss any aftershave that contains alcohol in the trash. Alcohol, while a germ-killing antiseptic, actually dries out the skin and increases the risk of irritation. After shaving, your skin craves moisture in order to repair itself. If you prefer to use an aftershave, pick up one that is alcohol- and fragrance-free, and full of skin-soothing and moisturizing ingredients.

Rose water

Natural rose water can serve as a gentle, calming aftershave and is a favorite among many shaving connoisseurs and barbers. Don't worry, the scent is usually light and doesn't smell girly.

Conditioner

If your beard is exceptionally coarse, using a bit of hair or beard conditioner will soften it right up to make it more touchable and inviting to others (see Resources).

Face wash

In most situations, your beard won't require a cleanser of its own. Your face wash will do just fine to keep it in fine condition. Use a gentle cleanser that's free of exfoliating bits that can irritate skin. Using a face wash before you shave is also a great way to prevent clogged pores and help soften the beard.

Exfoliant

Shaving is an efficient method of exfoliation. Each stroke of the razor takes a bit of skin along with the hair it slices. If you shave every day (or even five days a week), using any kind of exfoliant on your beard area is overkill for your skin. And please, don't exfoliate right before you shave or your skin will feel raw and irritated. If you don't shave every day, feel free to use a gentle exfoliant that contains gentle bits or beads instead of crushed shells or stones that can be way too aggressive on skin and cause trouble.

Mustache wax

If your style needs a little help in looking its best or defying gravity, pick up a high quality mustache wax that's non-comedogenic (meaning it won't clog your pores or cause acne break-outs). They come in different textures, fragrances, colors, and various levels of stiffness. Whether you hope to sport a gravity-defying style or you just want to keep your stache in place in windy conditions, a touch of wax can help. Try a few to find the one that gives you the hold and manageability you want. Men with longer Handlebar or Dali-style staches that require a little more molding and sculpting might prefer a stiffer wax, while guys who just want to hold the tips together will probably prefer a softer, more malleable formula.

Quick Tip: If you use a mustache wax that is not water-based and therefore difficult to remove, add shampoo to your beard or mustache while it is still dry. Oily waxes repel water, so by applying shampoo to a dry mustache, the shampoo will be able to break the bonds of the wax before you add the water.

Step by Step: The Perfect Shave

You might be thinking, "I know how to shave." Now think about all the ingrown hairs, the razor burn, irritation, and nicks you've inflicted upon yourself. Still feeling confident in your shaving skill?

Where did you learn to wield that razor you hold in your hand? Perhaps your father or granddad walked you through the motions as a young boy, or you read about it in a popular men's magazine. While shaving remains one of the oldest rituals among men—dating way back to the days of Egyptian pharoahs—many men still shave like they are hacking away at weeds.

If you learned to shave from your father, chances are that he taught you all the same bad habits he picked up from his father. Consider this your opportunity for razor therapy.

The best time to shave is during or immediately after a shower. The warm water and moisture softens hair and skin, allowing the blade to glide across your face with ease, minimizing irritation. If you can't shave then, wet a towel with warm water and apply it your face and neck for five minutes for the same effect.

1. Apply a pre-shave oil—especially if your skin is prone to irritation. Applying an oil before shaving will reduce friction and drag between the blade and your skin. It also helps to seal vital moisture in. Despite what you've heard, not all oils are bad for your skin. Pre-shave oils won't clog your pores or cause breakouts.

2. Lather up your favorite shaving cream or gel. No matter what dear old Dad said, foams aren't as good because of the large air bubbles that don't provide enough moisture and lubrication. Apply the cream or gel to your face in a circular motion to help lift whiskers and ensure even saturation. Over the last few years, classic badger hair shaving brushes have gained popularity. Badger hair retains moisture, provides mild exfoliation, and lifts whiskers while creating a rich lather—not to mention that it looks rather cool in your bathroom.

3. Determine the direction of your hair growth by dragging a finger up and down your face. Your beard will feel smooth when brushed in one direction (with the grain, the same direction as hair growth) and prickly in the opposite one (against the grain of its growth).

4. Using your hand, gently pull the skin on your cheek taut. This helps

to create a flat cutting surface for the blade. Doing so helps the blade do its job more efficiently.

5. Using a new, sharp blade and applying little to no pressure against your skin, drag the razor down your cheek in the same direction as your hair growth. Try not to go over the same area more than once or twice if possible. Fewer passes means fewer chances for irritation. Rinse your blade after every one to two passes to avoid clogs.

6. After shaving both cheeks, draw your upper lip over your teeth to create a flat shaving surface, and shave your mustache area in a downward direction. Repeat around your chin and lower lip area.

7. Shave your neck last because it will give the oil and shaving cream extra time to soften your skin and hair. The skin around the neck is more prone to irritation than your face. Pay close attention to the changes in the direction of hair growth on your neck. For most men, hair grows downward on the face and upward on the neck. But some unlucky men have hair that grows in all sorts of ways on the neck area.

8. If you're prone to five o'clock shadow and your skin isn't particularly sensitive to shaving, you may shave against the grain. (If your skin is easily irritated, avoid shaving against the grain and skip steps nine through eleven, below).

9. Before shaving against the grain, apply more pre-shave oil and shaving cream to your face to provide a moisturizing cushion between skin and blade.

10. Using gentle strokes, draw the razor in an upward direction on your cheek—against the growth of your beard. Repeat on the opposite cheek, upper lip, and chin.

11. When shaving against the grain on your neck, it's important to watch for any shifts in the direction of the hair growth. When in doubt, just brush your fingers over your beard to determine the direction of its growth.

12. After shaving, rinse your skin with cool water to close pores and reduce redness.

13. Using an alum block will immediately stop any bleeding and serve as a natural antiseptic to prevent infection.

14. Gently pat your skin dry with a clean towel.

15. Apply an oil-free moisturizer or alcohol-free aftershave. You can find all sorts, including unscented products and those for allergic or sensitive skin.

Harm Reduction

Shaving is a pain. For the clean-shaven man, the daily chore can feel like a Sisyphean exercise. You remove hair only to have it grow back, and then you do it again. For many men, this particular grooming routine causes all sorts of discomfort, from razor burn to ingrown hairs, nicks, and cuts. Here we'll help you tame the blade—but if you're still having trouble, ask a dermatologist.

Razor Burn

Razor burn is usually caused by friction between the blade and your skin. It's the post-shave irritation or rash. Luckily, it's easily remedied with a few high-quality products and extra attention to your shaving habits.

Apply a pre-shave oil before a shaving cream. The oil will further lubricate your skin and reduce friction between the blade and your skin.

Use a fresh blade. Replacement cartridges for your razor can be expensive, but shaving with a dull blade costs a lot more to your skin and appearance. Replace your blade every four to five shaves. Once your blade dulls, it becomes jagged and loses its high-tech coatings that also reduce friction.

Use a light touch. Pressing the razor too hard on your skin will increase the friction. Let the blade do the work and allow your hand to be the guide.

Make fewer passes. The more times you shave the same area, the more likely you will experience irritation. If you're using a five-blade cartridge and make two passes, it's the equivalent of going over the same spot ten times with a single blade.

Try a razor with fewer blades. Not everyone will benefit from the four- and five-blade models. Guys who are particularly prone to irritation should consider a two- or three-blade design.

Avoid shaving against the grain, that is, in the opposite direction of the hair growth.

Use a soothing moisturizer or aftershave that does not contain alcohol. Moisturizers help your skin heal and provide protection from the elements. Alcohol-based aftershaves will only further irritate your visage.

Ingrown Hairs

Ingrown hairs occur when a whisker grows into the skin. Sometimes it struggles to break through the skin barrier, or it grows out and curls back into the skin. These can cause scarring and razor bumps if not cared for properly. Men with curly hair (and those of African descent) are at particular risk for ingrown whiskers.

To treat an ingrown hair, dermatologists recommend using a pair of sanitized tweezers to lift the tip of the whisker out from underneath the skin. But be careful not to remove the hair entirely or you'll surely have another ingrown hair in the same place (see page 131). Once the tip is above the surface, you can trim the hair with scissors or shave it normally.

Here are a few tips for preventing ingrown hairs:

Avoid shaving against the grain. Shaving against the growth of the hair might provide a closer shave, but it can also cause ingrown hairs.

Use a "PFB" (Pseudofolliculitis barbae) razor (like Bump Fighter). Some razors are specially designed to fight ingrown hairs by not cutting as close; they leave whiskers just long enough to protrude from the skin.

Use a moisturizer after shaving. Regularly moisturizing your skin will keep it soft and help whiskers grow out easily.

Nicks and Cuts

Nicks and cuts usually occur when you're not paying attention, shaving too quickly, or using an old blade.

Take your time. Don't rush through shaving. Look at it as a moment of peace and quiet when you can truly take care of yourself. Taking slow, deliberate strokes with the razor will not only prevent cuts, but you'll enjoy a better quality shave because the blade will work more efficiently.

Avoid distractions. Don't multi-task while shaving. Don't answer your phone, talk to your wife or roommate, or rehearse your presentation for a morning meeting.

Take shorter strokes. If you try to shave your cheek, chin, and neck in one stroke, you're going to cut yourself. Divide your face into small areas with similar topography. When shaving areas with wild turns or bumps, use short strokes to make sure that you're holding the razor at the right angle throughout the full pass.

Use a new blade. An old, dull blade is more likely to cut you. The jagged edge tends to scrape more skin with each pass.

Try a razor with the blades closer together. With less space between the blades, skin is less likely to get caught between the blades.

Ask the Expert:

Bradford Katchen, MD, knows a thing or two about skin, facial hair, and looking your best. As a Manhattan-based cosmetic dermatologist, great skin is his business. He owns and operates SkinCareLab, one of NYC's best spas for men and women. Dr Katchen has cared for some of the world's most beautiful faces, including Hollywood stars, TV personalities, and models. Here, he offers wise words on how a beard can solve your skin woes, how to shave with acne, and why plucking ingrown hairs can lead to trouble.

Q. What are the risks of shaving when you have acne?

A. The most irritating type of acne is actively inflamed cystic acne. If you shave over an active infection, the acne can worsen and potentially scar. Also, acne medications such as Accutane and topical Retin-A can make shaving more difficult. Both make your skin dryer and prone to irritation.

Some people with active acne seem to have no problem shaving with cartridge razors (like a Mach 3 or Fusion) or electric shavers. Personally, I prefer cartridge razors since you can change the blade frequently and reduce the risk of spreading infection. But guys who cut themselves often may do better with an electric shaver.

Because bacterial infections of the hair follicle—known as folliculitis—often accompany severe cystic acne, maintaining a closely cropped beard can help. It allows the hairs to grow out from beneath the skin and reduces the risk of trauma from ingrown hairs or other irritations associated with shaving.

Q. How can people with acne can get a more comfortable shave?

A. The best time to shave is after a shower. Use a thick layer of protective shave gel or cream, make just one pass with the razor, and shave in the direction of your hair growth, not against it.

Q. If someone has acne, which shaving and aftershave products should they avoid?

A. Gels generally tend to be more hydrating than other shaving products. I prefer fragrance-free formulas for guys with very sensitive skin and active acne. Aftershave products should always be lightweight and oil-free and contain no alcohol. Alcohol can dry and irritate the skin.

Q. I get ingrown hairs on my neck all the time! What can I do to prevent new ones and treat what I have?

A. First of all, never pull them out! A hair that tends to grow inward will do it again. If you pull it out completely, you'll experience the same problem. It is best to allow the beard to grow, if possible. When you see the ingrown culprit, you can use tweezers to gently pull the tip of the hair from beneath the skin, but don't yank it out completely. Then go ahead and clip or shave it. Don't shave it too close, however, or it will go back beneath the skin. Allow a small amount of the whisker to remain visible above the skin.

Q. I wear a beard and mustache year round. I keep breaking out where my beard is long. What's causing this and how can I stop it?

A. If you're breaking out around a single hair, then it's probably folliculitis, a bacterial infection of the hair follicle. This can be treated with topical and/or oral antibiotics. Check with your dermatologist.

Sometimes the skin may simply be irritated and it's not acne at all. It could be seborrhea—dandruff that appears on the eyebrows and scalp and can also show up on beards. Seborrhea can be treated with antifungal or cortisone-based shampoos that are available over the counter or from a doctor.

Q. When I shave, I tend to break out. What am I doing wrong? Is it the products I'm using or my shaving technique?

A. It could be a combination of the two. That is why I suggest shaving after a shower, using a protective agent. Shave with a fresh, clean blade, and only shave once in one direction. Afterward, apply a lightweight lotion that is oil-free. If you shave in the morning, using a lotion with a sunscreen is even better.

Q. Which is better for my skin: shaving foam, shaving gel, shaving cream, or shaving soap?

A. I recommend shaving gels. I find them easier to work with, more hydrating, and more protective than foams. Some cream-based formulas clog the razor and make shaving less efficient.

Q. How can I reduce the itch associated with growing a beard?

A. The itch is probably caused by one of two things: either your beard hair is trying and failing to pierce your skin or it's rubbing on sensitive skin. Try a cream or lotion with an exfoliating ingredient such as glycolic or salicylic acid. These soften the skin and exfoliate the top layer so that hair can get through it more easily. It will also result in fewer ingrowns. Meanwhile, keeping your skin and hair well-moisturized will ease the irritation and itch.

The Classic Shave: Strop, Hone, Cup, Brush, Blade
Using a Shaving Brush

Classic shaving has swept back into fashion in the last decade. Men want to recreate the barbershop shave experience at home. Not only are guys signing up to learn how to use a classic straight-edge blade, but they are also exploring shaving accoutrements such as shaving brushes.

Long heralded for their ability to create luxurious lather, shaving brushes actually provide a great service to the daily chore. The bristles gently remove dry, dull skin from the face and also lift whiskers up and away from the face, allowing the razor to cut hair more efficiently with each pass.

Shaving brushes are typically crafted from badger hair for their natural ability to retain water. As a result, shaving brushes create a richer lather and continue to deliver moisture to the skin and hair—making it softer and easier for the razor to cut, resulting in a more comfortable shave.

Badger hair brushes come in four levels of quality determined largely by texture. Pure badger is the most affordable and the roughest. It is dark in color and typically comes from the underbelly of the beast. Best badger is slightly more expensive, softer, and is made from the hair that covers twenty to twenty-five percent of the badger's body. Super badger is very high quality and very soft and has a silvery or off-white color. The rarest and softest (read: most expensive) badger hair is called silvertip. The hair is taken from the badger's neck during the winter months when the tips of the hair becomes silvery.

Not all brushes are made from badger hair. Boar hair and synthetic versions are also available for a more affordable price, but they don't function as well as the real thing.

Step-by-Step
1. Fill your sink with hot water and soak the brush bristles for fifteen to twenty seconds or hold it under a running faucet.
2. While you might feel tempted to shake, tap, or wring out the water from the brush—don't. The more water in the brush, the better the lather it will produce, the softer your whiskers will become, and the better the shave you'll receive.
3. Place a quarter- or dime-sized amount of cream inside the heart of the brush. Gently close the bristles and submerge the brush in water for another ten to fifteen seconds, then start lathering by gently whisking the brush inside a shaving mug. If the foam is too wet or runny, remove the excess water from the brush by tapping it gently on the sink and try whisking again until you get a warm, fluffy lather.

If you prefer to go a little more old-school and use a shaving soap, the steps are slightly different.

1. Whisk the brush over the soap in a circular motion as though you were scrambling eggs. After fifteen to twenty seconds, the lather will become rich and primed for shaving.

2. Once you've worked up a rich lather, apply the brush to your face and spread the lather over your beard and mustache in circular motions. Apply enough pressure to lift whiskers away from your face, but don't push so hard that the bristles flatten against your face, or you'll miss out on the benefits of using a brush entirely.

3. If you need more lather during your shave, dip the brush in water and whip up some fresh foam.

4. Once you're done shaving, rinse the brush under warm water until all the cream or soap is free from the bristles. Tap the brush gently against the sink to get rid of excess water and hang the brush to dry on a handsome-looking stand.

Honing and Stropping

Some men love the whole shaving ritual so much that they want to celebrate it, even prolong it, rather than get it over with. That is what our great-granddaddies did long before disposable five-blades came along. Using and maintaining an open razor is a very traditional, masculine thing to do. Your face will never feel cleaner, smoother, or as vibrant as when you've had a close shave. You'll look and feel like a new man. Shaving like this is slow, deliberate, and requires both reflection and concentration. It's time for yourself; an act of self-care and pampering. The sensuous pleasures of the experience (touch, smell, sight) will get you off to a good start for a day filled with multi-tasking and electronic overload. You'll learn patience, precision, and pride in your top-notch appearance. Talk to your barber and ask him to coach you in the art and science of open razor shaving rituals. Ask him if he thinks you have the patience and coordination to carry the whole thing off. You can even ask him to supervise you for a trial run. Tip him double that day.

How to Hone a Razor

Hones are usually rectangular blocks made of abrasive material and are used for sharpening open razors. They often have a synthetic surface that helps produce a sharp edge, while natural-surface hones are better for producing fine, longer-lasting razor edges. Check the Resources at the end of the book for places you can buy a hone, and then follow the manufacturer's recommendations carefully. (No, you cannot sue if you chop off your fingertip.)

You can lubricate the hone's surface with oil or water. Then hold the razor with one hand and the hone block with the other. Position the razor flat against the hone in the upper right corner edge, facing inward. Carefully slide the blade diagonally and down across the hone. Use gentle pressure. Pass the blade from its heel to toe along the hone with the downward stroke. Rotate the blade so that the opposite edge is against the hone and pass it as above but from upper left to lower right corners of the hone.

Next, perform a reverse stroke, passing the blade along the hone from lower left to upper right and lower right to upper left corners. Gentle pressure should be applied as the blade is pushed upward. If you're clumsy, get your barber to show you how to use the thing properly. Utter the words "Jolly good!" as you complete the task.

How to Strop a Razor

A variety of strops are available. Barbers usually prefer hanging strops, which consist of a canvas side for cleaning the razor's edge and a leather side for achieving a smooth finish. You can certainly hang one of your own in your bathroom, as this will impress visitors.

Position the razor near the top of the strop with the cutting edge facing upward. Apply light pressure as you draw the razor across the strop. Pass the blade diagonally from heel to toe. Rotate the blade so that the cutting edge is pointing downward and then draw the blade upward to the top of the strop in a similar stroke. Do not apply pressure during this motion! Rotate the blade and continue to pass it up and down the length of the strop until the right sharpness for you has been achieved.

The Shave

Excerpted and reprinted with permission from *The Art of the Straight Razor Shave: A Basic Guide*, by **Christopher Moss**, a fifty-something English-born Nova Scotian curmudgeon who has always enjoyed wet-shaving. In his guide to straight razor shaving, he writes, "If you are the kind of guy who likes to work with your hands, to make things, who isn't afraid to change his own oil or a tire, who likes fountain pens over ballpoints, vinyl over compact disks, tubes over transistors, who likes his film cameras, and enjoys the smell of developer and fixer, who thinks muzzleloaders are way cooler than assault rifles, then it might just be the thing for you."

Hold the razor with your dominant hand. Put your thumb on the underside of the shank, your index, middle and ring fingers on top of it, and your little finger on the tang, so that the scales stick up between the ring and little fingers. Before the blade touches the skin, let's clear up a couple of things. The optimum angle between blade and skin is about thirty degrees—too little will pull on the hairs without cutting them, and too much will encourage the blade to dig in. The other thing is that the blade is safer when kept moving; it is sharp enough that if the edge is left on your skin in one spot, and the angle is too steep or the pressure used is too great, it will sink in. This is counterproductive, to say the least. So don't be afraid to move the blade on your face, but do be sure to move it in a direction at right angles to the edge, *never* sideways, or parallel to the edge of the blade. You will cut yourself this way. We will change hands for the other side of the face.

The easiest way to begin is to lay the razor flat on your cheek and then lift the spine slightly and straight away start moving down the cheek to shave the first pass. Use very little pressure. Be sure to use the fingers of your other hand to stretch the skin. This gives a smooth surface for the razor to glide over and reduces the chance of a cut, making the shave closer and more comfortable. I remember the tremor in my hand the first time I did this, but I knew it could be done, and indeed was done by every non-bearded man in the world at one time.

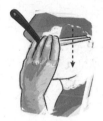 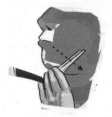 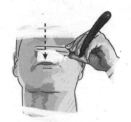

After completing the first pass, you should put the razor down and rinse the face with hot water from the sink. Then re-lather just as you did for the first pass. The second, across-the-grain pass requires a little more care, and you will know if your razor isn't sharp enough at this point; it will pull if it isn't. Assuming it is, proceed with the second pass. Try to lead with the point a little— if the razor is slightly oblique to the direction of travel, each hair will meet the blade at an angle which allows it to slide to the side a tiny bit, and thus the blade cuts it more easily as it slides along the edge in a tiny slicing action. If the razor seems to catch, don't keep on pushing it through, but lower the spine a little closer to the skin and then proceed. Here is the sequence for going across the direction of hair growth on my face:

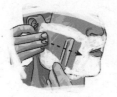
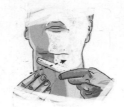
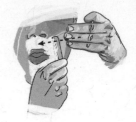

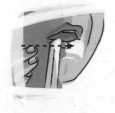

Notice how I am going upward on the sides of my neck; this is because the hair grows laterally here, so this is actually across the grain. Where the hair grows downwards under the chin, the razor is moved across it.

Once again, put down the razor and rinse and re-lather. The final pass requires a very light touch, and you must be aware of what the edge is doing at all times. Don't daydream or you will cut yourself. Remember to drop the spine if it seems to be catching; never push on through. Again lead with the point—the pictures show what I mean by this. The trickiest part of the face is under the chin, and with most of the hair gone in the first two passes this part should be easy on the third. I will be going against the direction of hair growth in these pictures, so the razor travels sideways toward the midline on my neck, upwards under the chin and on the face itself. On the upper lip I don't go directly against the grain, but obliquely upwards. Here it is:

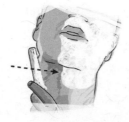
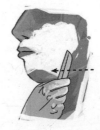

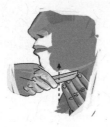 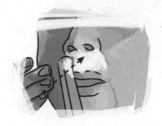

Notice the oblique upward stroke on the upper lip. There are bound to be a few tiny nicks after your first shave this way, so after the third pass put down the razor and splash very cold water onto your face to rinse off the remaining lather. The cold water will constrict blood vessels and halt most nicks from bleeding. A styptic pencil should be at hand for touching on those that aren't stopped. This stings for a moment but works well. You will rarely need it at all once you have the hang of it! Then pat your face dry with a towel.

Rinse your brush in cold water, then squeeze it to get most of the water out. Flick it vigorously to get the rest out. Either hang the brush up in a stand or simply stand it upright (if you have faith in your science lessons and understand that capillary action will keep the water remaining from sinking down into the knot of the brush). Rinse the razor under the hot tap, being very careful to avoid touching the edge against the tap or the sink. A ding of this kind is a major repair on a straight razor and you aren't ready to undertake that just yet! It doesn't matter too much whether you strop the razor now, or just before the next shave.

You did it! Hopefully you are still in one piece and not too weak at the knees.

Get a Professional Straight Razor Shave
by **Brett and Kate McKay**, a husband and wife team who run the Art of Manliness, a blog dedicated to uncovering the lost art of being a man. Reprinted with permission.

Maybe you've tried the straight razor at home and are convinced of its merits. Treat yourself to a professional job done by your trusty barber!

Why Get a Straight Razor Shave
It's relaxing. The straight razor shave is the facial for manly men. The experience is definitely a treat. There's nothing like a hot towel on your face or the masculine fragrance of shaving cream to sap the stress right out of your body. The few times I've gotten a straight razor shave, I've fallen asleep because it's so darn relaxing.

When you get a straight razor shave, you can almost feel the testosterone increasing in your body. It feels cool to be taking part in a ritual that thousands of men from history experienced. Plus, in a world where women are pretty much doing everything men are, a straight razor shave is one of the few activities that is still completely and exclusively male.

It's dangerous. At least it feels that way. There's nothing like letting another man hold a razor-sharp piece of metal to your neck to remind you that you're alive.

What to Expect from a Straight Razor Shave
The barbershops that I've been to charge twenty dollars for a straight razor shave. Some places will be more and some places may be less. But twenty dollars seems to be the going rate.

The two places I've gotten a straight razor shave had a pretty similar process. Here's how it typically goes. You'll sit in a cool barber chair, and the barber will tilt it back. He'll start off putting a nice hot towel around your face to soften up your whiskers. After the first hot towel, some barbers rub cleanser on your face to open up the pores and to make sure your face is nice and clean for a good shave. After that, another hot towel.

Next, they might put some conditioner on your whiskers to soften them up, followed by another hot towel.

Now it's on to the shaving cream. Most barbers have their own secret recipe for shaving cream that has been passed down for generations. The shaving cream will come from a heated dispenser. It feels really nice on your face.

They'll then take the razor to your face. Because of health codes, most barbers use disposable straight edge razors as opposed to traditional straight razors. Some men would argue that you'll notice the difference. Honestly, I haven't.

After a first pass with the razor, you'll get another hot towel. Shaving cream is reapplied, and another pass is made.

When the barber is done removing your beard, he'll give you a cold damp towel to close your pores and then splash on some manly smelling aftershave.

Bada bing! You just got a straight razor shave. You'll walk out of the barbershop feeling rejuvenated, relaxed, and uber-manly.

For our bearded brethren, have a professional trim and clean your beard up. I hear some barbers have some nice shampoos designed specifically for beards that smell particularly manly.

When to Start Over: Age and Facial Shape

Facial hair is a gift that keeps giving. You can grow, trim, and chop as long as you have "T" (testosterone) running through your veins and use fur (or smooth skin) to your advantage. Read this book over and over for inspiration (and check out our website) as you go.

A beard, sideburns, and mustache that look good on you at twenty may not look so hot once you reach middle age. You may have less hair on top, and wearing a long beard might make you look lopsided. Your face will lose fat and padding and as a result your nose may seem more prominent, something you want to conceal rather than celebrate. You might sprout an extra chin or two, or acquire scars or wrinkles and need a bit of camouflage. Facial hair may go gray and make you look older than you want to. If you put on weight, a mustache may make you look like Hardy (the fat one) from Laurel and Hardy. If your face gets thinner, you may end up looking like Abe Lincoln.

When at the gym, on the street, or at work, pay attention to men your age who wear facial hair. Look through popular magazines for actors you admire—Sean Connery has always used changing facial hairstyles to his advantage despite increasing baldness. Try one of the virtual photo-fur try-outs (see Resources). Ask your barber what he thinks of your current facial hair and how it might be made more flattering. Refer to the previous sections on choosing facial hair styles that flatter your aging face.

But please, don't look to your son or nephew for style cues.

Things evolve. Things change. Most of us will grow then shave then grow again. Fashion trends will come and go. You're free to follow them or buck them entirely. Don't be afraid to experiment and indulge your hirsute (or hairless) whims. Just remember: You are the master of your own follicular destiny. Go forth and grow wisely.

How to Tell If It's Time to Change Your Look

Fashion trends come and go at breakneck pace. Not long ago, the hairless metrosexual ruled supreme, but has now given way to today's more hirsute style. So how do you know if your current facial hair style has fallen from fashion? How do you know if you're a trendsetter or a holdover? Here are a dozen signs that it's time to change your look:

1. Mothers hide their children from you.

2. You are constantly selected for extra security screening at the airport.

3. Children write you letters with their Christmas lists, and you're always asked to play Santa Claus at the company holiday party.

4. People ask if the circus is in town.

5. Your grandfather wears the same style of facial hair.

6. Your dentist tries to swap styling tips with you.

7. Your optometrist suggests a much stronger prescription before he even checks your eyesight.

8. People refer to you as grandpa or daddy ... and you're only in your thirties.

9. People drop coins in your coffee cup when you sit in the park or wait for the bus.

10. Friends and family send you razors and shaving cream as gifts.

11. You still smell of the taco or curry you ate last week.

12. Your spouse or partner stops kissing you.

ARTICLES (IN PRINT)

Burns, Nick. "One Hairy Lip, A Mix of Messages." *The New York Times* (November 2, 2006), p. E3.

Cutler, Rodney. "How to Use Your Facial Hair." *Esquire* (May 2008), p. 50.

Martin, Peter. "Mind the Beard Line." *Esquire* (May 2008), p. 50.

Mulkeen, Martin. "Taming the Recession Beard." *Men's Journal* (June 2009), p. 66.

Schaefer, Kayleen. "The Best Straight-Razor Shaves on the Planet." *Details* (December 2006), p. 82.

Shaefer, Kayleen. "The Gentleman Spa." *Details* (October 2006), p. 300.

Staff. "Facial Fur Tache Back." *Esquire* (May 2009), p. 143.

———. "How to Care for Your Vacation Beard (No Matter How Long Your Vacation)." *Esquire* (Spring 2009), p. 104.

———. "Let It Grow, Man: Scruff Isn't Just for Porn Stars and Pirates Anymore." *Men's Health* (September 2006), p. 90.

———. "Men's Health Grooming Awards." *Men's Health* (May 2009), p. 136.

———. "Peach Fuzz Problems." *Maximum Fitness* (November/December 2008), p. 38.

———. "Sideburns: How Long Can You Go?" *Men's Health* (September 2006), p. 90.

———. "The Layoff Beard." *Details* (January/February 2009), p. 54.

———. "The Shaving of Whiskers." *Esquire* (March 2009), p. 58.

ARTICLES (ONLINE)

Alexander, Dave. "Tips on Caring for Your Beard: Advice for Maintaining Your Facial Hair," *About.com* [undated], *http://menshair.about.com/od/facialhair/a/beardcare.htm*

"All You Need to Know about Shaving Brushes, Sort of ..." *Perfect Shave*, August 8, 2009, *http://perfectshave.blogspot.com/2009/08/all-you-need-to-know-about-shaving.html*

Armitage, Tom. "Gillette Research Promotes Bare-faced Chic." *Cosmetics Design-Europe*, October 26, 2004, *http://www.cosmeticsdesign-europe.com/news/ng.asp?id=55669-gillette-research-promotes*

Babic, Balil, "Facial Hair Styling Tips." *Article Alley*, Sept. 20, 2005, *http://www.articlealley.com/article_9398_34.html*

Em & Lo, "Stubble Theory: What Your Facial Hair Is Really Saying." *New York Magazine*, August 6, 2006, *http://nymag.com/relationships/mating/18852/*

Kealy, Kat, "Playoff Beards and Other Thoughts." *Hockey Buzz.com*, April 7, 2008, *http://hockeybuzz.com/blog.php?post_id=14600*

Mapes, Diane, "Hairy Economy Trend: Beards are Back." MSNBC, February 10, 2009, *http://www.msnbc.msn.com/id/29108262/*

McGrath, Ben. "Dept. of Labor: Strike Beards." *New Yorker*, January 7, 2008, *http://www.newyorker.com/talk/2008/01/07/080107ta_talk_mcgrath*

"Playoff Beard." Wikipedia, *http://en.wikipedia.org/wiki/Playoff_beard*

Shelton, Karen Marie, "Men's Facial Hair: Mustaches Designs." Hair-Boutique.com, December 15, 2003, *http://www.hairboutique.com/tips/tips3907.htm*

Staff. "Celebrities with Moustache." *Men's Flair*, March 19, 2007, *http://www.mensflair.com/celebrity-styles/celebrities-with-moustache.php*

———. "Facial Hair Styles." *Men's Flair*, March 23, 2007, *http://www.mensflair.com/grooming-abcs/facial-hair-styles.php*

Vierra, Dan, "Mustaches Are Growing in Popularity." *Arizona Daily Star*, December 11, 2006, *http://www.azstarnet.com/allheadlines/159599*

Wilson, Eric, "Paul Bunyan, Modern-Day Sex Symbol." *The New York Times*, March 23, 2006, *http://www.nytimes.com/2006/03/23/fashion/thursdaystyles/23BEARDS.html?ei=5088&en=5a8*

BOOKS

Corson, Richard. *Fashions in Hair: The First Five Thousand Years*. London: Peter Owen Limited, 2000.

Dickson, E. Jane. *Debrett's Manners for Men: What Women Really Want*. Richmond, UK: Debrett's Limited, 2008.

Dunkling, Leslie and John Foley. *Guinness Book of Beards and Moustaches*. London: Guinness Publishing, 1990.

Editors of Esquire Magazine. *Esquire: The Handbook of Style: A Man's Guide to Looking Good*. New York: Hearst Books, 2009.

Estep, Keith. *Best of Shaving Mugs*. Atglen, PA: Schiffer Publishing, 2001.

Flocker, Michael. *The Metrosexual Guide to Style: A Handbook for the Modern Man*. Cambridge, MA: Da Capo Press, 2003.

Maggio, Carole. *Facebuilder for Men: Look Years Younger*. London: Pan Books, 2002.

Peres, Daniel. *Details Men's Style Manual: The Ultimate Guide for Making Your Clothes Work for You*. New York: Gotham, 2007.

Peterkin, Allan. *One Thousand Beards: A Cultural History of Facial Hair*. Vancouver: Arsenal Pulp Press, 2001.

Pinfold, Wallace. *A Closer Shave*. New York: Artisan, 1999.

Professional Services for Men: Facial Massage, Shaving and Hair Design Clifton Park, NY: Thomson Delmar Learning, 2007.

Trusty, L. Sherman. *The Art and Science of Barbering*. Los Angeles: Wolfer Printing, 1976.

Waters, David. *Grooming Essentials for Men*. London: Carlton Books, 2002.

Zaoui, Myriam and Eric Malka. *The Art of Shaving*. New York: Clarkson Potter, 2002.

MOVIES

Splitting Hairs, Firelight Films (2008).
The Glorius Mustache Challenge, Real Eyez Films (2007).

More references can be found at *www.beardedgentleman.com*

WEBSITES

Gillette: *www.gillette.com*
Photoshop Tutorials: Add Facial Hair: *ilike2photoshop.blogspot. com/2008/05/add-facial-hair.html*
Virtual Haircuts for Men: *www.hairfinder.com/computerhairstylesmale.htm*

JOIN THE CLUB: TWENTY TOP FACIAL HAIR CLUB AND CONTEST WEBSITES

Clubs
Belgium: Antwerp Moustache Club (Snorrenclub Antwerpen): *www. snorrenclubantwerpen.be/*
Canada: Beard Team Canada: *www.beardteamusa.org/canada.html*
England: Handlebar Club: *www.handlebarclub.co.uk/index.php*
England: British Beard Club: *thebritishbeardclub.org/*
France: Paris Moustache Club: *www.parismoustacheclub.com/*
Germany: Association of German Beard Clubs (Verband Deutscher Bartclubs): *www.verband-deutscher-bartclubs.de/vdbjoomla/*
Germany: Berlin Beard Club (1. Berliner Bartclub e.V.): *www.1-berliner-bart-club.de/Joomla/index.php*
Italy: International Moustache and Beard Club (International Club Baffi e Barbe): *baffomania.it/*
Norway: The Norwegian Moustache Club (Den Norske Mustaschklubben): *www.skippys.no/english/historikk.html*
Russia: Russian Beard Club: *www.borodatyh.net/*
Sweden: The Swedish Moustache Club (Svenska Mustaschklubben): *www.mustascher.se/*

Switzerland: Rhein Valley Moustache and Beard Club (Rheintaler Schnauzund Bartclub): *www.bart.li/startseitescbr.htm*
USA: National Beard Registry: *www.nationalbeardregistry.org*
USA: Beard Community: *www.beardcommunity.com*
USA: All About Beards: *www.beards.org*
USA: Organization for the Advancement of Facial Hair: *www.ragadio. com/oafh/*

Contests
World Beard and Moustache Championships: *www.akbeardclub.com/*
North American Beard and Moustache Championship: *www.nabmc. whiskerclub.org/*
Whiskerino: *www.whiskerino.org/2007/*
Wahl Nation: *www.wahlnation.com*

Best Beard (and Goatee) Sites
All About Beards: *www.beards.org/links.php*
Beards of Hollywood: *www.beardsofhollywood.com/Beard Stylings: www. beardstylings.com*
George Carrol: *georgecaroll.blogspot.com/2009/09/famous-whiskers.html*
Goatee.org: *www.goatee.org*
Half-Bakery: *www.halfbakery.com/idea/goatee_20templates*
Hudson's FTM Resource Guide: *www.ftmguide.org/facialhair.html*

Best Sideburn Sites
Hudson's FTM Resource Guide: *www.ftmguide.org/facialhair.html*

Best Mustache sites
American Mustache Institute: *www.americanmustacheinstitute.org/*
Handlebar Club: *www.handlebarclub.co.uk/index.htm*
Hudson's FTM Resource Guide: *www.ftmguide.org/facialhair.html*
Moustache Database: *www.moustache-database.freeservers.com/*
Mustache Aficionado: *www.mustachecentral.com/*

Mustache Summer: *www.mustachesummer.com/*

FORUMS AND GROUPS

Badger & Blade: *badgerandblade.com/*
The Beard Board: *jefffsbeardboard.yuku.com/*
Beard Community: *beardcommunity.com/*
Beard Team USA: *beardteamusa.org/*
Beards Are Not a Crime: *beardsarenotacrime.com/*
Beards BeCause: *beardsbecause.com/home/beards_because-home.php*
Beards for Cancer: *www.wastedapples.com/beardsLATEST.html*
Beards for Peace: *beardsforpeace.org/default.aspx*
Beards from Below: *beardsfrombelow.org/index.php*
The British Beard Club: *thebritishbeardclub.org/*
DMOZ (links): *www.dmoz.org/Arts/Design/Fashion/Hair/Facial_Hair/*
The Fabulous World of Beards and Mustaches: *worldofbeards.co.uk/*
High Sierra Whisker Club/Beard & Mustache Championships: *www.*
highsierrabeardandmoustache.com
Organization for the Advancement of Facial Hair: *www.ragadio.com/oafh/*
Shave Blog: *www.shaveblog.com*
Shave Den: *theshaveden.com/*
The Society of Bearded Gentlemen: *beardedgents.com/*
Society of Beards: *societyofbeards.com/*
Tennessee Beard & Mustache Club: *www.tennesseebeards.com/*
The Whisker Club: *whiskerclub.org/*
World Beard and Mustache Championships: *www.worldbeardchampion-*
ships.com/Support/clubs.htm

SHAVING PRODUCTS AND SUPPLIES

Acqua di Parma: *www.acquadiparma.it*

Alford & Hoff: *www.alfordandhoff.com*

American Crew: *www.americancrew.com*

Anthony Logistics: *www.anthony.com*

Appearances for Men: *www.appearancesformen.com*

Baxter of California: *www.baxterofcalifornia.com*

Beard Care: *www.beardcare.co.uk*

Biotherm Homme: *www.biotherm-usa.com*

Blademail: *www.blademail.com*

Charles Nicholls: *www.charlesnicholls.co.uk*

Clarins Men: *www.clarinsmen.com/*

ClassicShaving.com: *www.classicshaving.com*

Clinique Skin Supplies for Men: *www.skinsuppliesformen.com*

ConsumerSearch.com: *www.consumersearch.com//electric-shavers/reviews.
  html*

Dermalogica: *www.dermalogica.com*

Edwin Jagger: *www.edwinjagger.com*

Em's Place: *www.emsplace.com*

eShave: *www.eshave.com/*

Executive Shaving: *www.executive-shaving.co.uk*

Geo. F. Trumper: *www.trumpers.com/*

Great Razors: *www.greatrazors.com*

Grooming Lounge: *www.groominglounge.com/*

Jack Black: *www.getjackblack.com/*

Kiehl's: *www.kiehls.com*

Korres: *www.korres.com*

La Roche Posay XY Homme: *www.xyhomme.com*

Lab Series Skincare for Men: *www.labseries.com/*

Lee's Safety Razors: *www.leesrazors.com*

Malin + Goetz: *www.malinandgoetz.com*

Menscience Androceuticals: *www.menscience.com/*

Molton Brown: *www.moltonbrown.com/*

Nickel For Men: *www.nickel.fr*
Pacific Shaving Company: *pacificshaving.com*
QED USA: *www.qedusa.com*
Saint Charles Shave: *www.saintcharlesshave.com*
Sharps: *www.sharpsusa.com*
Shavemac.com: *www.shavemac.com*
Shaving Stuff: *www.shavingstuff.com/*
Straight Razor Designs: *www.straitrazordesigns.com*
Task Essential: *www.taskessential.com/*
Taylor of Old Bond Street: *www.tayloroldbondst.co.uk/*
The Art of Shaving: *www.theartofshaving.com/*
The Gentleman's Shop: *www.gentlemans-shop.com*
The English Shaving Company: *www.theenglishshavingcompany.com*
The Old'e English Shavingshop: *www.shavingshop.co.za*
The Well Shaved Gentleman: *www.thewellshavedgentleman.com*
Truefitt & Hill: *www.truefittandhill.com*
Vulfix Old Original: *www.vulfixoldoriginal.com*
Wahl: *consumer.wahl.com/*
Zirh: *www.zirh.com/*

THEATRICAL AND COSTUME FACIAL HAIR SUPPLIERS

Anytime Costumes: *www.anytimecostumes.com*
Broadway Costumes: *www.broadwaycostumes.com*
Buy Costumes: *www.buycostumes.com*
Costumes 4 Less: *www.costumes4less.com*
International Fun-Shop: *www.fun-shop.com*
Hollywood Toys & Costumes: *www.hollywoodtoysandcostumes.com*
Malabar: *www.malabar.net*
Mardi Gras Costume Shop: *www.mardigrascostumeshop.com*
Platinum Costumes: *www.platinumcostumes.com*

STYLES, TIPS, AND TECHNIQUES

About.com/Facial Hair Guide: *menshair.about.com/od/facialhair/Facial_Hair_Guide_for_Men.htm*

AskMen.com: *askmen.com/fashion/fashiontip_300/367b_fashion_advice.html*

Bigger Better Beards: *www.biggerbetterbeards.org/*

Jon Dyer's Blog: *www.dyers.org/blog/beards/beard-types/*

Men's Flair: *www.mensflair.com/grooming-abcs/designer-stubble.php*

Men's Health: *www.mh.co.za/style/grooming*

Nicks and Cuts at eHow.com: *www.ehow.com/how_116346_keep-shaving-nick.html*

Facial Hair Handbook: *www.facialhairhandbook.com and www.jackpassion.com*

Hairmixer: *www.hairmixer.com*

My Barber: *www.mybarber.com*

Remington: *www.remington-products.com/grooming/tips.htm*

Shave My Face: *shavemyface.com*

Straight Razor Place: *straightrazorplace.com*

"Beards" on Wikipedia: *en.wikipedia.org/wiki/Beard*

MISCELLANEOUS LINKS

Art of Manliness: *www.artofmanliness.com*

Beardie Weirdie Blog: *www.beardieweirdie.co.uk/blo*

Beard*Revue: *www.beardrevue.com*

Bearduary: *bearduary.com*

Beards & Baldies: *www.beardsandbaldies.com*

Fuck Yeah Beards: *fuckyeahbeards.tumblr.com*

New Yorker Cartoon Bank: *www.cartoonbank.com*; search "beard cartoons"

Off the Mark Cartoons: *offthemark.com/search-results/key/beards/*

Whiskerino: *www.whiskerino.org/2007/beards*

Year of the Beard: *www.yearofthebeard.com/?cat=6*

WHERE TO BUY GREAT SHAVING PRODUCTS

C.O. Bigelow: *bigelowchemists.com*
The online home for the famed NYC apothecary Bigelow Chemists.

Drugstore.com: *www.drugstore.com*
Everything in your drugstore … online. But they carry so much more than your Gillette shave gel and razor blades.

Grooming Lounge: *www.groominglounge.com*
These guys know grooming. The online home for the men's barbershops in Washington, DC, and Atlanta, they offer a wide selection of shaving implements and tonics at a great price.

Lee's Safety Razors: *www.leesrazors.com*
A fine selection of Dovo straight razors, strops, and Merkur Safety Razors for shaving enthusiasts.

MenEssentials: *www.menessentials.com*
Canada's online grooming headquarters. A well-edited selection of top grooming brands and equipment—including classic double-edged safety razors.

Nashville Knife Shop: *www.nashvilleknifeshop.com*
An exhaustive selection of Dovo straight razors, safety razors, strops, grooming implements, creams, potions, and tonics—even kitchen knives (hey, one-stop shop!).

Sephora: *www.sephora.com*
The mall mecca for skincare, fragrance, and products for women also carries a huge selection of products for guys. Don't expect to find replacement blades here, but shaving creams and aftershaves are plentiful.

SkinCareLab: *www.skincarelab.com*
This site, run by one of New York City's top celebrity dermatologists, doesn't offer shaving equipment but is full of great men's skincare and shaving products from foams and gels to aftershaves and more.

Space NK: *www.spacenk.com*
London's answer to Sephora carries a number of European brands that are difficult to find stateside.

LEARN MORE!

One Thousand Beards: *A Cultural History of Facial Hair* by Allan Peterkin (Vancouver: Arsenal Pulp Press, 2001). Contains over 200 additional book and web references (see also *www.arsenalpulp.com/1000beards*).

INDEX

About the Authors

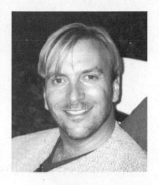

Allan Peterkin is the author of the bestselling *One Thousand Beards: A Cultural History of Facial Hair* and six other books on cultural history and medicine. His comments on facial hair have been published in *Esquire*, *Men's Health*, the *Wall Street Journal*, the *Financial Times*, the *New Yorker*, the *New York Times*, *Sports Illustrated*, *US*, and dozens of other international media outlets.

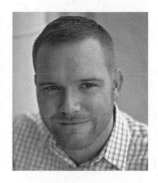

Nick Burns is an internationally published writer and journalist. Specializing in grooming, fashion, and health, he has contributed to the *New York Times*, the *Washington Post*, the *Wall Street Journal*, *New York Magazine*, *GQ*, *Details*, *Men's Journal*, *Elle*, *Out*, *Cargo*, *Health.com*, *Thomson Reuters*, and many more. *The Bearded Gentleman* is his first book.

Check out *www.beardedgentleman.com* for blogs, promotions, new links, and tips!